The ASQ:SE User's Guide

The ASQ:SE User's Guide

for the
Ages & Stages Questionnaires: Social-Emotional

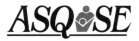

by

Jane Squires, Ph.D.

Diane Bricker, Ph.D.

and

Elizabeth Twombly, M.S.

Early Intervention Program
Center on Human Development
College of Education
University of Oregon, Eugene

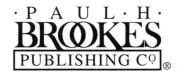

·P A U L·H·
BROOKES
PUBLISHING Cº ®

Baltimore • London • Sydney

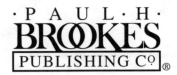

Paul H. Brookes Publishing Co.
Post Office Box 10624
Baltimore, Maryland 21285-0624

www.brookespublishing.com

Typeset by Barton Matheson Willse & Worthington, Baltimore, Maryland.

Manufactured in the United States of America by
Versa Press, East Peoria, Illinois.

All photographs in this book and on the cover are used by permission of the
individuals pictured or their parents and/or guardians.

The people, programs, and situations described in this book are completely fictional.
Any similarity to actual individuals or circumstances is coincidental, and no
implications should be inferred.

Ages & Stages Questionnaires (ASQ)™ is a trademark owned by
Paul H. Brookes Publishing Co. See the end of this guide for information about
accompanying products in the ASQ™ system.

Second printing, July 2003.

Library of Congress Cataloging-in-Publication Data

Squires, Jane
    The ASQ:SE user's guide : for the Ages & stages questionnaires, social-emotional : a
parent-completed, child-monitoring program for social-emotional behaviors / by Jane Squires,
Diane Bricker, Elizabeth Twombly.
        p.   cm.
    Includes bibliographical references and index.
    ISBN 1-55766-533-8
        1. Child development—Testing.   2. Infants—Development—Testing.   3. Child development
deviations—Diagnosis.   I. Bricker, Diane D.   II. Twombly, Elizabeth.   III. Squires, Jane. Ages
& stages questionnaires, social-emotional.   IV. Title: Ages & stages questionnaires, social-
emotional user's guide.   VI. Title: Ages and stages questionnaires, social-emotional user's guide.
RJ51.D48S64 2001
    155.4′028′7—dc21   2001035553

British Library Cataloguing in Publication data are available from the British Library.

Contents

ASQ:SE

List of Tables and Figures

ASQ:SE

APPENDIX B

APPENDIX D

About the Authors

The ASQ:SE system, including the *Ages & Stages Questionnaires: Social-Emotional*—English and Spanish versions—and *The ASQ:SE User's Guide,* was developed by the following authors:

Jane Squires, Ph.D., Associate Professor, Early Intervention Program, Center on Human Development, University of Oregon, Eugene, Oregon 97403

Dr. Squires is an associate professor in special education, focusing on the field of early intervention. She is also Associate Director of the University of Oregon Center for Excellence in Development Disabilities. Dr. Squires has directed several research studies at the University of Oregon on the *Ages & Stages Questionnaires* and the *Ages & Stages Questionnaires: Social-Emotional.* In addition, she has directed national outreach training activities related to developmental screening and the involvement of parents in the assessment and monitoring of their child's development. In addition to her interests in screening and tracking, Dr. Squires directs a master's-level early intervention/special education personnel preparation program and teaches courses in early intervention at the University of Oregon.

Diane Bricker, Ph.D., Director, Early Intervention Program, Center on Human Development, University of Oregon, Eugene, Oregon 97403

Dr. Bricker has focused her professional career on the development and study of assessment/evaluation systems and intervention approaches for young children with disabilities and those who are at risk for disabilities. She has also been instrumental in the development and implementation of graduate-level personnel preparation programs. These programs have produced professionals who are delivering quality services to thousands of young children and their families. Dr. Bricker has published extensively in the field of early intervention.

Elizabeth Twombly, M.S., Senior Research Assistant, Early Intervention Program, Center on Human Development, University of Oregon, Eugene, Oregon 97403

Ms. Twombly is a senior research assistant at the Early Intervention Program. She has coordinated research activities on the *Ages & Stages Questionnaires: Social-Emotional* and has been involved in several research studies on the *Ages & Stages Questionnaires.* In addition, Ms. Twombly provides training and technical assistance to agencies on a variety of topics including screening and child-find activities, social and emotional assessment of young children, and the inclusion of parents in service provision.

Suzanne Yockelson, Ph.D., Research Associate, Early Intervention Program, Center on Human Development; and Program Coordinator, Educational Studies: Educational Foundations, and Instructor, Teacher Education Program, College of Education, University of Oregon, Eugene, Oregon 97403

Dr. Yockelson earned her doctorate at the University of Oregon in 1999. She consults with various state programs on using the *Ages & Stages Questionnaires* for developmental screening of infants and young children. She teaches courses on child development, research, and curriculum at the University of Oregon's College of Education. Dr. Yockelson's research interests include the social and emotional development of infants and young children and parent education.

Maura Schoen Davis, Ph.D., Early Intervention Program, Center on Human Development, University of Oregon, Eugene, Oregon 97403

Dr. Davis received her doctorate from the University of Oregon. Her dissertation investigated the interrater reliability and concurrent validity of the *Ages & Stages Questionnaires: Social-Emotional.* She has a master's degree in school psychology and has worked in early intervention and early childhood special education since 1991. Her research interests include screening and assessment of very young children.

Younghee Kim, Ph.D., Associate Professor, Master of Arts in Teaching Program, Education Department, Southern Oregon University, 1250 Siskiyou Boulevard, Ashland, Oregon 97520

Dr. Kim works with Early Childhood and Elementary Education Master of Arts in Teaching Program students at Southern Oregon University. She graduated from Sogang University in Seoul, Korea, in 1985. She received her master's degree in 1992 and her doctorate in 1996 from the University of Oregon in the area of early intervention/early childhood special education. Her special research interests include alternative assessment for young children with special needs, parent involvement in early intervention, and young children with emotional and social challenges, as well as multicultural education for children with diverse backgrounds. She lives with her husband and two young, bilingual children in Ashland, Oregon.

Preface

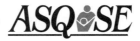

We began the development of the *Ages & Stages Questionnaires: Social-Emotional* (ASQ:SE) at the insistence of early intervention and early childhood service providers who regularly called and wrote, requesting that we expand the *Ages & Stages Questionnaires* (ASQ; Bricker, Squires, & Mounts, 1995; Bricker & Squires, 1999) to include social and emotional areas. These practitioners had no screening tools for assessing social and emotional problems in very young children and yet were required to identify children whose social-emotional competence was in doubt. Practitioners using the ASQ appreciated its parent-friendly format, clear assessment and scoring procedures, and psychometric integrity. They repeatedly asked if we could make a similar tool focused on social-emotional development. Could we develop a parallel parent-completed tool that measured social and emotional behaviors?

We appreciated the challenges faced by Early Head Start home visitors, Healthy Start home visitors, Head Start teachers, and early childhood personnel to accurately screen infants, toddlers, and young children to ascertain who would benefit from a follow-up in-depth evaluation in the area of social-emotional development. It seemed to us that an ASQ-like screening tool would be of great assistance to these teachers, home visitors, interventionists, and other child care workers.

We began with the realization that developing a screening tool for the social-emotional domains would be challenging. We were aware of the complexities involved in accurate assessment of social and emotional competence due to environmental, cultural, individual, and family variables. When is the crying of a 3-year-old "too much"? Are Fred's tantrums out of control, or are they within what is expected for a 2-year-old? Is it appropriate for Rhan, a 4-year-old, to constantly cling to her mother and have difficulty separating each morning at child care?

While most developmental skills—such as those included in the ASQ—can be reliably assessed (i.e., the child does the behavior currently or the child does not), atypical social-emotional behaviors are often more difficult to identify. We were unsure that a tool could be developed that objectively and clearly targeted behaviors that can vary according to setting, observer, child variables (temperament, health), cultural and family expectations, and social mores. Nonetheless, this seemed a challenge worth exploring.

Development of the ASQ:SE was rooted in our firm belief that parents can be accurate assessors of their young children's behaviors and development. The strong conviction that most parents can accurately evaluate their child's behaviors provided the necessary foundation for us to undertake this important task. Also compelling to us was the knowledge that the same needs that provided the impetus for the development of the ASQ remained. That is, parents and family members need to be genuinely involved in the assessment, intervention, and evaluation; tests and procedures were needed to monitor the development of infants at high risk for developmental problems because of medical, biological, or environmental factors or a combination; and resources remained limited and there continued to be pressure to find effective yet economical means to serve growing numbers of children who are at risk.

Our work in developmental screening made us aware of the growing need to examine and assess the social and emotional competence of infants and preschool children. The numbers of children who are living in poverty and who are more likely to show signs of anxiety, depression, and antisocial behavior are growing (Aber, Jones, & Cohen, 2000; Children's Defense Fund, 2001). Brain research has revealed the interplay between early brain development and the quality of environmental experiences (Shore, 1997) and has shown the huge impact that environmental experiences have on the developing structure of the brain (Nelson & Bosquet, 2000; Shore, 1997). We began development of the ASQ:SE system in 1996. As part of a doctoral seminar in the Early Intervention Program at the University of Oregon, we read widely and across disciplines about social and emotional competence and disability. The variety of approaches, definitions, and philosophies that we found was staggering.

In line with our philosophical views, a transactional approach to development (Sameroff, 2000; Sameroff & Chandler, 1975), with an ecological emphasis (Bronfenbrenner, 1977), formed the conceptual underpinnings for the ASQ:SE. The social learning model (Bandura, 1977; Patterson, Reid, & Dishion, 1992), which posits that social learning occurs as a function of the child's daily social interactions, was also deemed important. In addition, the developmental organization theory of Cicchetti (1993) and the marginal deviation model (Dishion, French, & Patterson, 1995; Reid, 1993) provided useful complements. These models established that disturbances or inappropriate social learning at earlier levels will likely cause continuing and more serious disturbances at later ages. Finally, developmental theory (Fischer & Rose, 1994; Gesell, 1933; Piaget, 1950) provided the foundation for the range and span of behaviors.

As a result of our literature review, a series of questions appropriate to infants (6 and 12 months), toddlers (18 and 24 months), and children (30, 36, and 48 months) was generated that parents and caregivers could read and understand. Questions were grouped into the areas of self-regulation, compliance, communication, adaptive behaviors, autonomy, affect, and interactions with people. The format of the ASQ was followed as closely as possible. However, different answering and scoring formats were adopted that better fit the assessment of social-emotional competence. The questions were compiled into a tool initially called the *Behavior-Ages & Stages Questionnaires* (B-ASQ; Squires, Bricker, Twombly, Yockelson, & Kim, 1996). The B-ASQ was piloted with more than 800 parents and providers at numerous sites, including Healthy Start in Hawaii, Early Head Start of Southern Oregon, and Oregon Migrant Head Start. (Acknowledgments to individuals and programs instrumental in the development of the ASQ:SE follow this preface.) After 2 years of gathering field data, in 1999 the B-ASQ was renamed the *Ages & Stages Questionnaires: Social-Emotional.* As part of the revision, some items were omitted and others revised. A 60 month interval was also added. From the beginning of the project, we sought and incorporated feedback from parents and service providers. We believe this feedback has been vital to the successful development and testing of the ASQ:SE.

Psychometric studies based on more than 3,000 questionnaires (described in Appendix A) suggest that most parents and caregivers can use the ASQ:SE accurately to provide initial screening information. Finding external support for the development and study of the ASQ:SE has been almost as challenging as developing the tool. For the most part, we have had to rely on the good faith of practitioners and parents who thought our work important; practitioners and parents completed the ASQ:SE with little or no remuneration. We have included a formal "thank you" to many of these individuals in the acknowledgments. It is only because of this support and conviction that we have been able to pursue our work.

The ASQ:SE includes eight intervals covering the 3- to 66-month age span that can be used individually or as a series. Scoring options include *most of the time, sometimes, rarely or never,* and a column for parents/caregivers to check if the item is a concern. Cutoff points were empirically derived based on ASQ:SE scores on these 3,000-plus questionnaires. Children whose scores are on or above the cutoff points should be considered for further evaluation or referral for services; those with scores below the cutoff point can be monitored using another ASQ:SE in 6 or 12 months. Research is continuing on this screening tool; adjustments or changes in cutoff points will be posted on the Paul H. Brookes Publishing Co. web site (http://www. brookespublishing.com/asqse).

We are hopeful that the expansion of the ASQ system will improve the screening and tracking efforts of programs throughout the United States and elsewhere. Photocopying is permitted according to the following guidelines:

Purchasers of the **Ages & Stages Questionnaires: Social-Emotional (ASQ:SE): A Parent-Completed, Child-Monitoring System for Social-Emotional Behaviors** *are granted permission to photocopy the questionnaires as well as the sample letters and forms in* **The ASQ:SE User's Guide for the Ages & Stages Questionnaires: Social-Emotional: A Parent-**

Completed, Child-Monitoring System for Social-Emotional Behaviors *in the course of their agency's service provision to families.* Each branch office that will be using the ASQ:SE system must purchase its own set of original questionnaires; master forms cannot be shared among sites. The questionnaires and samples are meant to be used to facilitate screening and monitoring and to assist in the early identification of children who may need further evaluation. Electronic reproduction of the questionnaires is prohibited, and none of the ASQ:SE materials may be reproduced to generate revenue for any program or individual. Photocopies may only be made from an original set of color-coded master questionnaires and/or an original ***User's Guide.*** Programs are prohibited from charging parents, caregivers, or other service providers who will be completing and/or scoring the questionnaires fees in excess of the exact cost to photocopy the master forms. Likewise, the ASQ:SE materials may not be used in a way contrary to the family-oriented philosophies of the ASQ:SE developers. *Unauthorized use beyond this privilege is prosecutable under federal law.* You will see the copyright protection line at the bottom of each form.

For other questions pertaining to the ASQ:SE, please contact the Rights Department, Paul H. Brookes Publishing Co., Post Office Box 10624, Baltimore, MD 21285-0624, USA; 1-410-337-9580.

Early identification of children with social and emotional difficulties is of paramount importance for improving outcomes for children and families. Improved screening procedures that involve parents and caregivers should result in improved early identification procedures and more timely referral to intervention for children and families.

Jane Squires, Ph.D.
Diane Bricker, Ph.D.
Elizabeth Twombly, M.S.

REFERENCES

Aber, J.L., Jones, S., & Cohen, J. (2000). The impact of poverty on the mental health and development of very young children. In C.H. Zeanah (Ed.), *Handbook of infant mental health* (2nd ed., pp. 113–128). New York: Guilford Press.

Bandura, A. (1977). *Self-efficacy: The exercise of control.* New York: W.H. Freeman.

Bricker, D., & Squires, J. (with Mounts, L., Potter, L., Nickel, R., Twombly, E., & Farrell, J.). (1999). *Ages & stages questionnaires (ASQ): A parent-completed, child-monitoring system* (2nd ed.). Baltimore: Paul H. Brookes Publishing Co.

Bricker, D., Squires, J., & Mounts, L. (with Potter, L., Nickel, R., & Farrell, J.). (1995). *Ages & stages questionnaires (ASQ): A parent-completed, child-monitoring system.* Baltimore: Paul H. Brookes Publishing Co.

Bronfenbrenner, U. (1977). Toward an experimental ecology of human development. *American Psychologist, 32,* 513–531.

Children's Defense Fund. (2001, January 5). *Child welfare and mental health division* (Online). Available: www.childrensdefense.org/news_stats.htm

Cicchetti, D. (1993). Developmental psychology: Reactions, reflections, projections. *Developmental Review, 13,* 471–502.

Dishion, T., French, D., & Patterson, G. (1995). The development and ecology of antisocial behavior. In D. Cicchetti & D. Cohen (Eds.), *Developmental psychopathology: Vol. 2. Risk, disorder, and adaptation* (pp. 388–394). New York: John Wiley & Sons.

Fischer, K.W., & Rose, S.P. (1994). Dynamic development of coordination of components in brain and behavior: A framework for theory. In G. Dawson & K.W. Fischer (Eds.), *Human behavior and the developing brain* (pp. 3–66). New York: Guilford Press.

Gesell, A. (1933). Maturation and patterning of behavior. In C. Murchison (Ed.), *A handbook of child psychology.* Worcester, MA: Clark University Press.

Nelson, C.A., & Bosquet, M. (2000). Neurobiology of fetal and infant development: Implications for infant mental health. In C.H. Zeanah (Ed.), *Handbook of infant mental health* (2nd ed., pp. 37–59). New York: Guilford Press.

Patterson, G.R., Reid, B., & Dishion, T.J. (1992). *Antisocial boys.* Eugene, OR: Castalia.

Piaget, J. (1950). *The psychology of intelligence.* Madison, CT: International Universities Press.

Reid, J. (1993). Prevention of conduct disorder before and after school entry: Relating intervention to developmental findings. *Developmental and Social Psychology, 5,* 241–260.

Sameroff, A.J. (2000). Ecological perspectives on developmental risk. In J.D. Osofsky & H.E. Fitzgerald (Eds.), *WAIMH handbook of infant mental health: Vol. 4. Infant mental health in groups at high risk* (pp. 1–33). New York: John Wiley & Sons.

Sameroff, A.J., & Chandler, M.J. (1975). Reproductive risk and the continuum of caretaking casuality. In F.D. Horowitz, M. Hetherington, S. Scarr-Salapatek, & G. Siegel (Eds.), *Review of child development research* (Vol. 4, pp. 187–244). Chicago: University of Chicago Press.

Shore, R. (1997). *Rethinking the brain: New insights into early development.* New York: Families and Work Institute.

Squires, J., Bricker, D., Twombly, E., Yockelson, S., & Kim, Y. (1996). *Behavior-Ages & Stages Questionnaires.* Eugene: University of Oregon, Center on Human Development.

Acknowledgments

ASQ:SE

As with the *Ages & Stages Questionnaires*, the development of the *Ages & Stages Questionnaires: Social-Emotional* (ASQ:SE) evolved through a group effort. In particular, we thank Maura Schoen Davis, Pat DeMeurers, Younghee Kim, Susan Stewart, and Suzanne Yockelson, participants in an Early Intervention Program doctoral seminar. During the seminar, the initial review of the literature was conducted and the embryonic form of the questionnaires was constructed. In addition, Jane Farrell and LaWanda Potter participated in the initial development, and Deborah Eisert and Peggy Veltman, who are specialists in early development, helped us select the behavioral domains to be targeted by the questionnaires.

As with the developmental phase, many individuals assisted in data collection efforts. We would like to acknowledge Kimberly Murphy for her help in recruiting families and in organizing and maintaining data collection and data management systems. Robin High guided our data analysis efforts with care and competence. We would also like to acknowledge Kay Heo, who is now a professor at Woosuk University in South Korea, who made a significant contribution with her doctoral research on the initial version of the 24 and 36 month ASQ:SE intervals. James Jacobson and Karen Lawrence provided clerical and technical support.

In addition, we have received valuable feedback about the questionnaires from parents and caregivers as well as professionals in programs who have volunteered to use the ASQ:SE. In particular, we would like to thank Gladys Wong and the Healthy Start of Hawaii home visitors for piloting an early version of the ASQ:SE and sharing important feedback and data. Redmond Reams and his staff at the Children's Assessment Services at the Morrison Center in Portland, Oregon, have also assisted with data collection. Other programs in Oregon, including Migrant Head Start, Healthy Start, and Southern Oregon Early Head Start, have provided us with valuable feedback and data.

Thousands of families have completed ASQ:SE on their infants and young children and have been willing to participate a variety of interviews and assessments. These children and families have provided the necessary data to complete psychometric studies of the questionnaires. Other individuals and programs who assisted with data collection efforts are included in this list:

Nola Aichele, Yakima, WA
Mary Anderson, Pensacola, FL
Karen Athing, Upper Lake, CA
Pam Bauchwitz, Fort Walton Beach, FL
Jody Beck, Sandpoint, ID
Ginger Benson, Salem, OR
Julie Betts, Manassas, VA
Dana Brynelson, Vancouver, BC, Canada
Dina Calibeo, Taylor, MI
Judi Cameron, Eugene, OR
Sister Barbara Cline, Grand Rapids, MI
Jean Clinton, Bend, OR
Clyde Connolly, Arcata, CA
Dianne Crabtree, Shelton, WA
Theresa Constans Daly, New Orleans, LA
EC CARES, Eugene, OR
Evelyn Egan, Albuquerque, NM
Family Building Blocks, Salem, OR
Joan Firestone, Waterford, MI
Kim Gillis, Bonifay, FL
Jeff Goldblatt, Lansing, MI
Deborah Greenwald, Pensacola, FL
Hilary Hannon, Arlington, VA
Arlene Harmon, Kailua-Kona, HI
Amy Hayden, Urbana, IL
Stephanie Hodson, Kansas City, KS
Jackie Hogan, Kansas City, KS
Carole Hutchings, Williams Lake, BC, Canada
Ann Johnson, San Marcos, TX

Scynthia Jomini, Kimitat, BC, Canada
Margaret Kapun, Tyndall Air Force Base, Panama City, FL
Geri Lawrence, Milton, FL
Cory Leaphart, Pullman, WA
Jenny Lefeldt, Taylor, MI
Betty Lindstrom, Eugene, OR
Marti Loftus, Waterford, MI
Pat Malane, Barrie, ON, Canada
Maureen Markey, Portland, OR
Marilyn McGrath, Santa Monica, CA
Molly McGrath, Chicago, IL
Victoria Morrison, Panama City, FL
Juvata Nelson, Eugene, OR
Sue Nelson, Lewiston, ID
Ida Nissen, Pensacola, FL
Robin Patterson, Knoxville, TN
Redmond Reams, Portland, OR
Relief Nursery of Eugene, OR
Linda Richard, Phoenix, AZ
Elizabeth Rodriguez, Forest Grove, OR
Debbie Rossler, Bend, OR
Donna Schnitker, Burns, OR
Mara Stein, Lansing, MI
Willie Stevens, Winston-Salem, NC
Sandra Van Horn, Bradenton, FL
Judy Wendling, Upper Lake, CA
Annie Wolverton, Burnaby, BC, Canada
Bonita Young, Traverse City, MI

We give special thanks to Melissa Behm at Paul H. Brookes Publishing Co. for her many years of support and assistance. Jessica Allan, Dennis Hockman, Mika Sam, and Lisa Yurwit have ably assisted with ASQ:SE efforts.

The investment of time and effort by the many individuals we have named moved the ASQ:SE from a promise to a reality. Each has our thanks.

Jane Squires, Ph.D.
Diane Bricker, Ph.D.
Elizabeth Twombly, M.S.

1

Overview

ASQ:SE

A major obstacle to the delivery of appropriate early intervention services is the timely identification of infants and young children who are experiencing developmental problems. Timely identification requires establishing comprehensive child-find programs and monitoring systems and using economical, valid, and culturally sensitive assessment tools to deal effectively with the increasing numbers of children identified as at risk for developmental delays resulting from medical and environmental factors. One economical and effective option for timely identification is to involve parents as first-level screeners of their young child's development.

To meet the need for a parent-completed, first-level screening measure, the *Ages & Stages Questionnaires (ASQ): A Parent-Completed, Child-Monitoring System* (Bricker, Squires, & Mounts, 1995) was developed; in 1999 a second, expanded edition (Bricker & Squires, 1999) was released. The ASQ is a set of 19 questionnaires designed to identify infants and young children who show potential developmental problems. The questionnaires are designed to be completed by parents[1] when a child is 4, 6, 8, 10, 12, 14, 16, 18, 20, 22, 24, 27, 30, 33, 36, 42, 48, 54, and 60 months of age. They can be used individually (e.g., just the 16 month questionnaire) or in combination (e.g., the 4, 8, 12, and 16 month questionnaires) depending on the needs of the child and the resources of the program. Children are identified as needing further testing and possible referral to early intervention services when their ASQ scores fall below designated cutoff points.

Each ASQ questionnaire features 30 developmental items that are written in simple, straightforward language. The items are divided into five areas: communication, gross motor, fine motor, problem solving, and personal-social, with an Overall section addressing general parental concerns. The reading level of each questionnaire ranges from fourth to sixth

---

[1]Throughout this book and in the *Ages & Stages Questionnaires: Social-Emotional* themselves, "parents" is used to refer to individuals central to a child's life, including parents, grandparents, and other primary caregivers.

grade, and illustrations are provided when possible to assist with the understanding of items. For the 30 developmental items, parents check *yes* if their child performs the specified behavior; *sometimes*, indicating an occasional or emerging response; or *not yet*, indicating the child does not yet perform the behavior. Program staff convert each response to a point value, total these values, and compare the totals with established screening cutoff points. For detailed information on the ASQ, see *The ASQ User's Guide* (Squires, Potter, & Bricker, 1999).

RELATIONSHIP BETWEEN THE ASQ AND ASQ:SE

The *Ages & Stages Questionnaires: Social-Emotional (ASQ:SE): A Parent-Completed, Child-Monitoring System for Social-Emotional Behaviors* was developed to complement the ASQ by providing information specifically addressing the social and emotional behavior of children ranging in age from 3 to 66 months. Like the ASQ, the ASQ:SE is composed of a series of simple-to-complete questionnaires designed for use by a child's parents or other primary caregivers. The ASQ:SE is a screening tool that identifies infants and young children whose social or emotional development requires further evaluation to determine if referral for intervention services is necessary. The ASQ:SE focuses on a child's social and emotional behavior and therefore should be used in conjunction with the ASQ or another screening measure that provides information on a child's communicative, motor, problem-solving, and adaptive behaviors.

ASQ:SE USER'S GUIDE PURPOSE

The purpose of this user's guide to the *Ages & Stages Questionnaires: Social-Emotional* is to provide potential users of the ASQ:SE a rationale for the importance of examining the social and emotional competence of infants, toddlers, and preschool-age children. The guide also provides a detailed description of the questionnaires, which are designed to offer an accurate and low-cost method of screening young children for their emotional and social competence.

The ASQ:SE can be used in comprehensive Child Find systems to screen large groups of children for the early detection of potential developmental or emotional problems. Procedures for developing comprehensive Child Find systems that address recruitment, large-scale screening, and follow-up and referral activities are described later in this guide. The ASQ:SE Child Find system has three components: 1) planning the screening system, 2) conducting the screening system, and 3) following up the screening, as shown in Figure 1.

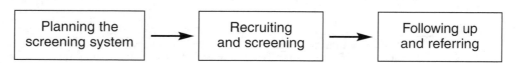

Figure 1.   Components of the ASQ:SE Child Find system.

An important feature of a comprehensive Child Find system is that it addresses the range of development in infants and young children. Screening groups of young children for social or emotional problems without also examining their cognitive, communicative, and motor behavior will likely yield, at best, an incomplete, and at worst, an inaccurate picture of the children's behavioral repertoires. Again the ASQ:SE should be used in conjunction with developmental screening tools that provide information on general child functioning in communication, motor, and cognitive areas.

INTRODUCTION TO THE ASQ:SE

Critical to the well-being of children is their ability to successfully regulate their emotions and manage their social interactions in ways that are acceptable to themselves and others. Children who manage their emotional and social behavior well are deemed competent, while those whose social or emotional behavior is inappropriate and unacceptable to others in their home or community are seen as troubled or "disabled." A growing body of evidence suggests that habituated and ingrained social and emotional problems are highly resistant to change and indeed are likely to intensify over time (e.g., Feil, Walker, & Severson, 1995; Sprague & Walker, 2000). Consequently, the early identification of social and emotional problems in infants, toddlers, and young children is essential if we are to assist them in building their emotional and social competence and reduce the likelihood of placement in special education programs, residential treatment, or later incarceration.

The need for prevention or early elimination of social or emotional problems in young children is an international concern, addressed in the United States by the Individuals with Disabilities Education Act (IDEA) Amendments of 1997 (PL 105-17). The timely identification of young children who have social or emotional problems or who are on a behavioral trajectory that will lead to problems with self, peers, and parents has proven to be challenging (Guralnick, 1997; Osofsky & Fitzgerald, 2000; Zeanah, 2000). Accurate, affordable strategies for the detection of social or emotional problems in young children have been particularly difficult to develop; consequently, the assessment of social and emotional competence of young children is often left undone until problems reach catastrophic levels requiring huge expenditures of intervention resources.

DEFINING SOCIAL AND EMOTIONAL COMPETENCE

As noted by Raver and Zigler (1997), there is a growing need to examine young children's emotional and social competence; however, defining and accurately measuring social and emotional difficulties in young children is a complex undertaking. Accurate assessment is complex because the parameters of acceptable behavior are influenced by age (e.g., it is acceptable for an infant to cry when hungry, but not for an 8-year-old child under most circumstances), by cultural and family values (e.g., some families/

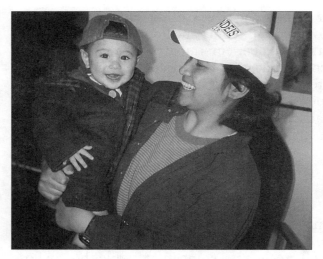

cultures encourage children to be active inquisitors, while others do not), and by environmental circumstances (e.g., it is generally acceptable to yell and run on the playground, but it is not acceptable to do so in most stores). The complexities inherent in defining appropriate social and emotional behaviors for children at different developmental levels lead to significant variability in what individuals, families, and communities identify as acceptable or tolerable. Behavior occurs on a continuum. It is often not clear to peers, siblings, or adults when a child's behavioral response has crossed the line from an appropriate but immature response (e.g., sucking one's thumb) or temporary misbehavior (e.g., an infrequent temper tantrum) to a repeated behavior (e.g., physically attacking other children) that will lead the child to serious difficulties. Descriptions of young children who have serious social or emotional problems suggest a gradual acceleration in either frequency of troubling behavior, severity of the behavioral response, or both, until the child crosses a line that at least some social partners deem unacceptable.

The complexities surrounding the definitions of social competence and emotional competence likely explain, in part, the lag in the timely identification of these problems in comparison with the more accurate and timely identification of cognitive, communication, and motor problems in young children (Bost, Vaughn, Washington, Cielinski, & Bradbard, 1998; Greenspan & Wieder, 1993; Zeanah, 2000; ZERO TO THREE, 1994). Our past inability to reliably identify children who require immediate intervention or those who are at significant risk for the development of serious social and emotional problems is particularly troublesome given the broad agreement that early identification of social or emotional problems or potential problems is the most effective prevention/intervention strategy that exists (Hart & Risley, 1995, 1999; Kazdin, 1987; Walker, Irvin, & Sprague, 1997; Walker et al., 1998).

The conceptual underpinnings for the ASQ:SE include the social learning model (Bandura, 1997; Patterson, Reid, & Dishion, 1992), which posits that social learning occurs as a function of the child's daily social interactions. In addition, the developmental organizational theory of Cicchetti (1993) and the marginal deviation model (Dishion, French, & Patterson, 1995; Reid, 1993) provide useful complements to the social learning theory. These theories suggest that deviation from normal developmental trajectories occurs when the important social, emotional, cognitive, and social-cognitive processes are not meaningfully integrated into more advanced levels of complex functioning. Disturbances (or inappropriate social learning) at earlier levels will likely cause continuing and more serious disturbances (faulty learning) at subsequent levels.

The IDEA Amendments of 1997 require the use of assessment procedures that address children's social competence and emotional competence as well as delays and disabilities; however, as Wittmer, Doll, and Strain have noted, "Comprehensive definitions of social and emotional competence and disability are not included in either federal or state statutes or regulations" (1996, p. 301). This deficit has likely been the impetus for a growing literature whose purpose is to understand and appreciate social and emotional development and what constitutes competence and disability (Fox, 1994).

Social competence and emotional competence are clearly connected; however, we and others believe that the constructs of social competence and emotional competence represent distinct though overlapping developmental areas and behavioral processes. Grappling with definitional problems associated with social and emotional behavior has concerned a number of important contributors to developmental psychology (e.g., Bost et al., 1998; Campos, Mumme, Kermoina, & Campos, 1994; Emde, Korfmacher, & Kubicek, 2000; Raver & Zigler, 1997; Thompson, 1994; Waters & Sroufe, 1983). From these authors' writings, two important working assumptions can be gleaned. The first assumption is that the constructs of the behavioral domains of social competence and emotional competence can be usefully separated into two areas, with the understanding that there is also overlap, in order to have a comprehensive and detailed understanding of young children's behavior. The second assumption is that definitions of these constructs need to address setting/time, developmental, individual, and family/cultural variables in order to be useful. That is, definitions composed of specific behaviors (e.g., child shares toys with peers) cannot adequately account for wide variations in social and emotional competence. Rather, definitions need to address general processes that transcend setting, developmental, individual, and family/cultural variables, and accommodate wide variation in specific behavioral indices. The definitions of social competence and emotional competence and their relationship are shown in Figure 2.

As shown in Figure 2, *social competence* can be defined as an array of behaviors that permits one to develop and engage in positive interac-

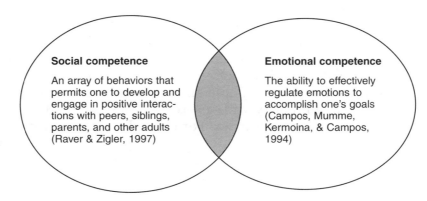

Figure 2.   Relationship between the behavioral domains of social and emotional competence.

tions with peers, siblings, parents, and other adults (Raver & Zigler, 1997). For example, four-year-old José, who typically engages and maintains his siblings and peers in appropriate play, elicits helpful assistance from teachers and parents, and uses positive strategies to solve problems, will likely be seen as a socially competent child. Four-year-old Linda, who typically fights over toys, is noncompliant, and attempts to solve problems by hitting, may not be seen as socially competent or at least may be seen as less socially competent than José.

Determining if children similar to José are socially competent is often more straightforward than determining social incompetence in children such as Linda. For example, when 3-year-old Tommy yells and snatches a toy, this social behavior may be deemed appropriate if the toy was originally taken from Tommy or inappropriate if Tommy instigated the aggression. When children exhibit prosocial behavior, the analysis is generally simple and straightforward; however, when children behave negatively, aggressively, or inappropriately, one *cannot* automatically conclude that the response indicates social or emotional incompetence or a problem.

Using a definition that transcends specific behaviors, *emotional competence* can be defined as the ability to effectively regulate emotions to accomplish one's goals (Campos et al., 1994). Emotional reactions can occur alone or overlay other responses. For example, if a toy is taken from Yolinda, she can cry or she can cry while delivering the verbal message, "Give it back." The 3-year-old who calms easily after a frightening experience, who controls his or her anger when disciplined, and who smiles and laughs at funny stories is likely to be seen as emotionally competent. The 3-year-old who cries uncontrollably at an unfamiliar sight, who screams frequently, and who is unresponsive for extended periods may be seen as emotionally troubled. As with social behavior, however, the appropriateness of an emotional response is affected by setting/time, developmental, health, and family/cultural variables. As with the definition of social competence, it is generally easier to decide if a child is emotionally competent than to decide if a child is emotionally troubled and in need of intervention.

ASSESSING SOCIAL AND EMOTIONAL COMPETENCE

Setting/time, development, health, and family/culture are four variables that should be addressed in assessing social and emotional competence. Setting/time variables can affect the interpretation of children's behavior. Children's behavior is often very different across different environments (e.g., home, school). These differences are due to the child's level of comfort and familiarity with a setting as well as the result of how the environment shapes behavior. For example, a parent who responds to a tantrum by giving the child attention may be reinforcing that behavior and causing tantrums to occur more frequently, and with increasing intensity, in the home setting. The same behavior, ignored at school, may quickly disappear. When a behavior occurs is also telling. For example, laughing when peers are enjoying an activity is far different from laughing when another child is seriously hurt. Acting shy and not participating in activities in the first week of school is quite different from not participating in the middle of a school year.

Second, the emotional and social competence of children must be viewed through a developmental lens. That is, the developmental level of children has a significant bearing on what other people in their environment find acceptable or unacceptable. For example, a toddler who cries when confronted by a stranger may be seen as normal by most adults who understand that the child is passing through a developmental stage. Most adults do not find it troubling when a 6-month-old pulls hair but will likely object to the same behavior exhibited by a 3-year-old. For most of us, it is unacceptable for an 8-year-old to snatch a toy from a peer, while we may tolerate such behavior from a 2-year-old. A 4-year-old who has a cognitive delay may appear noncompliant because she does not understand what is being asked of her. Ruling out a developmental delay is an important first step when interpreting young children's social-emotional behaviors.

Health variables, a third factor to consider, may also affect the interpretation of a child's social competence or emotional competence. Factors such as chronic illness (e.g., asthma, otitis media) need to be ruled out as well as variables such as whether the child has not had enough sleep, is hungry, or is reacting to a medication. A baby who has been fussy and difficult to soothe and who does not appear to be happy may well be suffering from an illness. A child who comes to school tired and hungry may display behaviors that are alarming but may merely need more sleep and food.

Finally, a child's social and emotional responses are clearly shaped by family values and culture. Some families/cultures place great importance on children being quiet and unobtrusive, while other families/cultures encourage active participation. Consequently, a quiet or verbally outspoken child may not be socially incompetent but may be behaving in ways consistent with family values. The interactions among family members, especially a child's relationship to his or her parents, play an important part in the development of social and emotional competence. For example, the interpretation of Sara's crying when approached by her stepfather would change if one knew that he often threatens to hit Sara. Some examples of family and cultural variables include family dynamics, cultural norms, and the primary language spoken by family members.

The four classes of variables just discussed are summarized in Table 1. Also listed are examples of questions that should be asked when addressing each variable. As indicated in Table 1, it is important to assess the child's social or emotional responses in reference to setting/time variables (e.g., Does the child act the same way at home and in child care? Is the setting unfamiliar?). In addition, the developmental age of the child is fundamental to determining whether the child's responses are acceptable, unacceptable, or fall in the questionable range. To the extent possi-

Table 1.   Classes of variables and associated questions to consider when assessing social and emotional competence in infants, toddlers, and preschool-age children

Variable	Assessment questions
Setting/time	Where, when, and under what environmental conditions does the behavior occur?
Development	What is the child's developmental level?
Health	What is the child's health status?
Family/cultural	What family/cultural factors are potentially associated with the behavior?

ble, the assessment should also address health variables (e.g., past health history, current status, day-to-day well-being). Finally, the assessment should be sensitive to and take account of family/cultural variables (e.g., Does the family/culture value "quiet" children? Does the child speak and understand English and Mandarin? What is the child's relationship to his or her parents?).

Assessments of children's social and emotional behavior require definitions that treat the areas separately but also appreciate the overlapping and interactive nature of these domains, as previously shown in Figure 2. For purposes of assessment, *social competence* can be defined as the child's ability to use a variety of communicative and interactive responses to effectively manage his or her social environment. Children's social competence is developmentally grounded in that both the maturity of the responses and external expectations for the child's responses change over time. *Emotional competence* is defined as the managing or regulating of one's emotional responses to obtain desired goals in ways that are acceptable to others. As with social competence, emotional competence is a developmental phenomenon that is expected to change and mature over time. Also important to note is that emotional development in young children is affected by environmental feedback (e.g., providing verbal feedback, setting expectations) just as with other developmental processes (Thompson, 1994).

The ASQ:SE was created using these definitions of social competence and emotional competence. Because the ASQ:SE is a screening tool, it does not address all of the assessment questions listed in Table 1. The primary purpose of the ASQ:SE is to assist parents and early intervention and early childhood personnel in the timely identification of children with responses or patterns of responses that indicate the possibility of their developing future social or emotional difficulties. In other words, the ASQ:SE is designed to identify children whose social competence or emotional competence differs in some way from expectations. The ASQ:SE is not a diagnostic tool for identifying children with serious social or emotional disorders; rather it should be seen as an aid in identifying young children who may benefit from more in-depth evaluation and/or preventive interventions designed to improve their social competence, emotional competence, or both.

2

Description and Design of the ASQ:SE

ASQ:SE

NEED FOR THE ASQ:SE

There is a significant need for a psychometrically sound, low-cost screening instrument that can accurately reflect the emotional and social competence of infants, toddlers, and preschool-age children. Table 2 presents a list of instruments frequently used to examine social and emotional competence in infants and young children. This table provides each instrument's name, author(s), publisher, year of copyright, age range, administration time, number of items, administrator, psychometric data, and its appropriateness as a screening tool. The data presented in Table 2 were taken from the instruments' test manuals or articles published by the instruments' authors.

A review of the information contained in Table 2 finds few instruments that cover the age range of 6 months through 6 years. Many of the tools listed in Table 2 were not designed for large-scale screening and, therefore, do not meet the criteria for low-cost screening. That is, the instruments listed take considerable time to complete, scoring is complex, and the interpretation of results must be done by highly trained professionals. In addition, many of the tools have limited data available on their reliability, validity, and utility. Finally, some of the instruments do not include the parent in a meaningful capacity.

The ASQ:SE was designed specifically as a low-cost screening instrument. Using the ASQ:SE is economical because it relies on parents to complete simple, easy-to-read questionnaires on their child at designated age intervals from 6 through 60 months. This approach automatically ensures meaningful participation by parents. Parents report that the questionnaires take little time to complete (i.e., 10–15 minutes). Scoring the questionnaires is simple and can be done by paraprofessionals. Interpreting the results is straightforward, as children's scores can be compared with empirically derived cutoffs that indicate if a child should receive further evaluation. The normative group closely approximates the 2000 United States census data (Bureau of the Census, 2001) for income, level of education, and ethnicity and includes a minimum of 175 cases at each

Table 2. Description of selected social-emotional assessment instruments

Name	Author(s) and copyright year (if available)	Publisher	Age range	Administration time	Number of items	Administrator	Psychometric data	Appropriate for screening
Ages & Stages Questionnaires: Social-Emotional (ASQ:SE)	Jane Squires, Diane Bricker, & Elizabeth Twombly (2002)	Brookes Publishing Co. Post Office Box 10624 Baltimore, MD 21285-0624 800-638-3775	6–60 months	10–15 minutes	Varies	Parent	Limited	Yes
Behavioral Assessment of Baby's Emotional and Social Style (BABES)	Karen M. Finello & Marie K. Poulsen (1996)	California School of Professional Psychology–Los Angeles 1000 South Fremont Avenue Alhambra, CA 91803 818-284-2777	Birth–36 months	10 minutes	29	Parent	Limited; under development	Yes
Behavioral Assessment System for Children (BASC)	Cecil Reynolds & Randy Kamphaus (1992)	American Guidance Service 4201 Woodland Road Circle Pines, MN 55014 800-328-2560	4–18 years	Varies	5 components	Parent or teacher	Yes	No
Carey Temperament Scales (CTS)	William Carey & Sean McDevitt	B-DI (Behavioral-Developmental Initiatives) 14636 North 55th Street Scottsdale, AZ 85254 800-405-2313	1 month–12 years	25 minutes	5 scales	Parent	Limited	No
Child Behavior Checklist for Ages 1½–5 (CBCL)	Thomas Achenbach & Leslie Rescorla (2000)	Achenbach System of Empirically Based Assessment (ASEBA) Room 6436	1½–5 years	10–15 minutes	100	Parent	Yes	No
Child Behavior Checklist for Ages 4–18 (CBCL)	Thomas Achenbach (1991)	1 South Prospect Street Burlington, VT 05401-3456 800-656-8313	4–18 years	10–15 minutes	113	Parent	Yes	No
Conners' Rating Scale–Revised	C. Keith Conners (1997)	Multi-Health Systems, Inc. 908 Niagara Falls Boulevard North Tonawanda, NY 14120 800-456-3003	3–17 years	10 minutes	Parent Scale (long form): 80 Teacher Scale (long form): 59	Parent Teacher	Limited	Yes
Devereux Early Childhood Assessment Program (DECA)	Devereux Foundation (1998)	Kaplan Companies PO Box 609 Lewisville, NC 27023-0609 800-334-2014	2–5 years	10 minutes	37	Parent	Yes	Yes
Early Coping Inventory (ECI)	Shirley Zeitlin, G. Gordon Williamson, & Margery Szczepanski (1988)	Scholastic Testing Services 480 Meyer Road Bensenville, IL 60106 630-766-7150	4–36 months	Varies; child observed across settings	48	Teacher, psychologist, and/or parent	Limited	No
Early Screening Project (ESP)	Hill M. Walker, Herbert H. Severson, & Edward Feil (1995)	Sopris West 4093 Specialty Place Longmont, CO 80504 303-651-2829	3–5 years	Stage 1: 1 hour Stage 2: 1 hour Stage 3: 40 minutes	Varies according to stages	Teacher Counselor Parent	Yes	Yes

Instrument	Author	Publisher/Contact	Age Range	Time	Number of Items	Administered by		
Eyberg Child Behavior Inventory (ECBI)	Sheila Eyberg	Psychological Assessment Resources, Inc. Post Office Box 998 Odessa, FL 33556 800-331-8378	2–16 years	10 minutes	36	Parent	Limited	Yes
Functional Emotional Assessment Scale (FEAS)	Georgia DeGangi & Stanley Greenspan (2000)	Appendix B in DeGangi, G. (2000). *Pediatric Disorders of Regulation in Affect and Behavior*. San Diego: Academic Press; for more information, call 301-320-6360.	7 months–4 years	15–20 minutes	6 versions; 27–61 items	Professional	Yes	Yes
Infant-Toddler and Family Instrument (ITFI)	Sally Provence & Nancy H. Apfel (2001)	Brookes Publishing Co. Post Office Box 10624 Baltimore, MD 21285-0624 800-638-3775	6 months–3 years	Varies	35 in interview; 38 in concerns checklist	Professional with parent	No	Useful in gathering preliminary information or as clinical tool
Infant-Toddler Social and Emotional Assessment (ITSEA)	Margaret J. Briggs-Gowan & Alice S. Carter	Not published commercially; contact the authors at 203-764-9093 for more information.	12–36 months	40 minutes	200	Parent	Yes	No
Infant/Toddler Symptom Checklist	Georgia DeGangi, Susan Poisson, Ruth Sickel, & Andrea Santman Wiener (1999)	Therapy Skill Builders 3830 East Bellevue Tucson, AZ 85716 800-872-1726	7–30 months	10 minutes	57	Parent	Limited	Yes
Parenting Stress Index (PSI), Third Edition	Richard R. Abidin	American Guidance Service 4201 Woodland Road Circle Pines, MN 55014 800-328-2560	Birth–12 years	20–30 minutes	120	Parent	Yes	No
Preschool and Kindergarten Behavior Scale (PKBS)	Kenneth Merrell (1994)	PRO-ED 8700 Shoal Creek Boulevard Austin, TX 78757	3–6 years	8–12 minutes	76	Parent and teacher	Yes	Yes
Social Skills Rating System (SSRS)	Frank M. Gresham & Stephen N. Elliott	American Guidance Service 4201 Woodland Road Circle Pines, MN 55014 800-328-2560	3–18 years	15–25 minutes	89	Parent and teacher	Yes	Yes
Temperament and Atypical Behavior Scale (TABS)	Stephen J. Bagnato, John T. Neisworth, John Salvia, & Frances M. Hunt (1999)	Brookes Publishing Co. Post Office Box 10624 Baltimore, MD 21285-0624 800-638-3775	11–71 months	5 minutes 15 minutes	Screener: 15 Assessment Tool: 55	Parent Professional	Preliminary	Yes
Vineland Social-Emotional Early Childhood Scale (SEEC)	Sara Sparrow, David Balla, & Dominic Cicchetti (1998)	American Guidance Service 4201 Woodland Road Circle Pines, MN 55014 800-328-2560	Birth–5 years, 11 months	15–20 minutes	Varies	Professional	Yes, but based on 1984 data	No

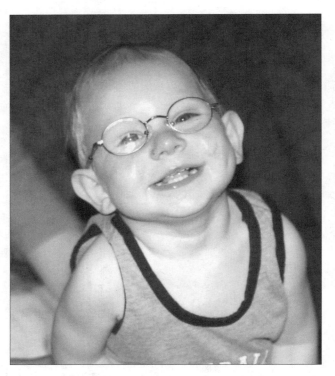

age interval. In addition, the reliability (e.g., interrater, test–retest, and internal consistency) and validity (e.g., concurrent) of the ASQ:SE have been studied with large groups of children. The underreferral (i.e., children who should be identified are missed) and overreferral (i.e., children are identified who should not be) rates for the ASQ:SE are acceptable, indicating that in most cases the instrument will accurately identify children in need of further evaluation (i.e., sensitivity) and those who do not (i.e., specificity). For more details on the psychometric properties of the ASQ:SE, see Appendix A in this *User's Guide.*

The most effective use of any screening instrument is within a larger, coordinated child-find system and not as an isolated activity; therefore, in addition to describing the ASQ:SE, procedures for developing a comprehensive community-based screening program are included later in this *User's Guide.*

DESCRIPTION OF THE ASQ:SE

The ASQ:SE is a series of eight questionnaires designed to be completed by parents to address the emotional and social competence of young children. The ASQ:SE has separate questionnaires for 6, 12, 18, 24, 30, 36, 48, and 60 month age intervals. Each questionnaire can be used within 3 months (for the 6 through 30 month intervals) or 6 months (for the 36 through 60 month intervals) of the chronological age targeted by the questionnaire. For example, the 6 month ASQ:SE can be used with infants from 3 through 8 months, the 12 month ASQ:SE with infants from 9 through 14 months, the 48 month questionnaire with children from 42 through 53 months, and the 60 month questionnaire with children from 54 through 65 months. Questionnaires vary in length, depending upon the age of the child. The number of questions per age interval is shown in Table 3.

Table 3.   Number of scored ASQ:SE items by age interval

	ASQ:SE age interval							
	6	12	18	24	30	36	48	60
Number of items	19	22	26	26	29	31	33	33

Table 4.   The ASQ:SE's seven behavioral areas and associated definitions

Behavioral area	Associated definition
Self-regulation	Items address the child's ability or willingness to calm or settle down or adjust to physiological or environmental conditions or stimulation.
Compliance	Items address the child's ability or willingness to conform to the direction of others and follow rules.
Communication	Items address the child's ability or willingness to respond to or initiate verbal or nonverbal signals to indicate feelings, affective, or internal states.
Adaptive functioning	Items address the child's success or ability to cope with physiological needs (e.g., sleeping, eating, elimination, safety).
Autonomy	Items address the child's ability or willingness to self-initiate or respond without guidance (i.e., moving to independence).
Affect	Items address the child's ability or willingness to demonstrate his or her own feelings and empathy for others.
Interaction with people	Items address the child's ability or willingness to respond to or initiate social responses to parents, other adults, and peers.

To the extent possible, the ASQ:SE items were written with an eye toward the setting/time, developmental, health, and family/cultural variables listed previously in Table 1 in Chapter 1. Although not specifically identified on the questionnaires, the item content of the questionnaires addresses seven behavioral areas: self-regulation, compliance, communication, adaptive functioning, autonomy, affect, and interaction with people. A list of these seven behavioral areas and their associated definitions are contained in Table 4. The separation into seven areas as well as the area names (e.g., self-regulation) is somewhat arbitrary but may help providers understand the organization of the ASQ:SE and the intent of individual questions.

Table 5 presents the seven behavioral areas, their associated general content indicators, and the specific items by ASQ:SE age interval. A review of Table 5 indicates that items are not evenly distributed across areas. In addition, the number of items and the content of items change over age intervals to accommodate changes in development.

The questionnaires have a standard format. There is a title page for each interval, followed by a sheet for recording name, date, address, and other identifying information. There is also a summary page at the end of each interval for programs to compile results and referral decisions. Each questionnaire item is followed by a series of three columns that parents can use to indicate whether their child does the behavior *most of the time, sometimes,* or *never or rarely.* A fourth column permits parents to indicate with a check if the behavior is of concern to them. Items on each questionnaire are coded Z, V, or X to permit quick and error-free scoring. Parents' responses are transferred to point values of 0, 5, or 10, respectively. Scores for each item are then combined into a total score. A high total score is indicative of problems, while a low score suggests that the child's social and emotional behavior is considered competent by his or her parent. Children whose total score exceeds the established cutoff

Table 5.   Behavioral areas, associated content, and specific items by ASQ:SE age interval

Behavioral area	Associated content	ASQ:SE age interval							
		6	12	18	24	30	36	48	60
Self-regulation	Can calm down	8	10						
	Body relaxed	10	8	5	4				
	Has trouble falling asleep	16	15	13	16				
	Calms down within time period	1	5	7	8	15	5	4	5
	Cries for long periods of time; screams, has tantrums	9	9	9	11	10	19	8	9
	Hurts others		21	25	25	28	29	31	30
	Has perseverative behaviors			11	21	11	21	22	22
	Is more active than peers					8	12	16	16
	Can settle down after excitement					9	7	7	7
	Stays with activities					12	13	18	13
	Moves from one activity to next					23	8	20	20
	Destroys and damages things					25	24	25	25
Total number of self-regulation items per interval		5	6	6	6	9	9	9	9
Compliance	Follows simple directions/ routine; follows rules			19	18	21	18	24	24
	Does what you ask					13	11	13	15
Total number of compliance items per interval		0	0	1	1	2	2	2	2
Communication	Listens; turns to look, smiles; looks	5	20	1	1	1	1	1	1
	Babbles		16						
	Lets you know/uses words when hungry, sick, tired	6	19	18	19	20	17	17	18
	Uses words for feelings						25	19	19
	Follows when you point			16	15	18			
Total number of communication items per interval		2	3	3	3	3	3	3	3
Adaptive functioning	Has trouble sucking	11							
	Stays awake for hour or longer during day	15							
	Takes longer than 30 minutes to feed	12	12						
	Is constipated or has diarrhea	18	18	17	17				
	Has eating problems	14	14	12	13	16	15	11	12
	Sleeps x hours in 24-hour period	17	17	15	14	19	16	15	17
	Hurts self on purpose			23	23	26	22	23	23
	Stays away from danger					24	23	26	26
	Has interest in sex						30	32	32
	Stays dry during day; is toilet trained							10	11
Total number of adaptive functioning items per interval		6	4	4	4	4	5	6	6
Autonomy	Checks when exploring; explores new places			21	20	22	20	21	21
	Clings to you more than you expect					3	4	2	2
Total number of autonomy items per interval		0	0	1	1	2	2	2	2

Note: Numbers in unshaded boxes indicate item number on the specific ASQ:SE questionnaire.

Behavioral area	Associated content	ASQ:SE age interval							
		6	12	18	24	30	36	48	60
Affect	Likes to be picked up and held; likes to be hugged and cuddled	3	4	6	7	2	2	5	3
	Stiffens and arches back	4	6	8	9				
	Is interested in things around her		11	10	10	14	10	9	10
	Seems happy					5	9	14	8
	Shows concern for others' feelings							28	27
Total number of affect items per interval		2	3	3	3	3	3	4	4
Interaction with people *Parents and other adults*	Smiles; smiles and laughs	2	1	3	3				
	Watches, listens; plays peek-a-boo; likes stories	7	7	22	22	6			
	When you leave, cries more than an hour			2	5				
	Enjoys mealtimes together	13	13	14	12	17	14	12	14
	Plays near; greets; talks to adults		3	20	6	4	3	3	4
	Looks for you; is too friendly with strangers		2	4	2	7	6	6	6
Peers	Likes to be around other children; plays alongside			24	24	27			
	Names a friend; takes turns and shares						26	27	31
	Other children like to play with your child						27	29	28
	Your child likes to play with other children						28	30	29
Total number of interaction with people items per interval		3	5	7	7	5	6	6	6
General concerns and comments	Anyone has expressed concerns about child	19	22	26	26	29	31	33	33
	Has concerns about child's eating and sleeping	20	23	27	27	30	32	34	34
	Has any worries about child	21	24	28	28	31	33	35	35
	Things you enjoy about child	22	25	29	29	32	34	36	36
Total number of general concerns and comments items per interval		4	4	4	4	4	4	4	4
Total number of all items per interval		22	25	29	29	32	34	36	36

points should be referred for a diagnostic evaluation. *This scoring pattern is the opposite of that of the ASQ, on which low scores, or the absence of developmental skills, indicates referral for further assessment.*

The ASQ:SE contains items related to competence and to problem behaviors. Examples of competence-related items include "Is your baby able to calm himself down (for example, by sucking on his hand or pacifier?)"; "Does your child like to be picked up and held?"; and "Does your baby let you know when she is hungry, hurt, or wet?" Examples of items related to problem behaviors include "Does your child have eating problems such as stuffing foods, vomiting, or eating nonfood items?" and "Does your child hurt himself on purpose?" Throughout the questionnaires, male and female pronouns are alternated by item. The questionnaires are also available in Spanish.

Each questionnaire can be completed by parents in 10–15 minutes, depending on the length of the questionnaire and the time it takes for individual parents to read and mark the appropriate answers. Reading level is approximately fifth- to sixth-grade level. As with any parent-completed assessment tool, not all parents will be able to read, understand, and accurately complete the ASQ:SE. For parents who do not read English or Spanish at a fifth- to sixth-grade level, the questionnaires can be used as an interview tool. For parents with cognitive and emotional disabilities, a professionally administered tool may be more appropriate. Cultural and ethnic variability will also need to be considered when using the ASQ:SE. If an item on the questionnaire is not appropriate for a family, it should be omitted. If an item is omitted, scoring procedures will need to be adjusted, as specified in Chapter 4 of this *User's Guide.*

OVERVIEW OF PSYCHOMETRIC DATA ON THE ASQ:SE

Validity, reliability, and utility studies were conducted on the ASQ:SE between 1996 and 2001 in order to determine the psychometric properties of the screening instrument. Normative studies included 3,014 preschool-age children and their families, distributed across the eight age intervals from 6 months through 60 months. Internal consistency, measured by Cronbach's coefficient alpha, ranged from .67 to .91, indicating strong relationships between questionnaire total scores and individual items. Test–retest reliability, measured as the agreement between two ASQ:SE questionnaires completed by parents at 1- to 3-week intervals, was 94%. These results suggest that ASQ:SE scores were stable across time intervals.

Concurrent validity, as reported in percentage agreement between ASQ:SE and concurrent measures, ranged from 81% to 95%, with an overall agreement of 93%. Sensitivity, or the ability of the screening tool to identify those children with social-emotional disabilities, ranged from 71% to 85%, with 78% overall sensitivity. Specificity, or the ability of the screening tool to correctly identify those children without social-emotional delays, ranged from 90% to 98%, with 95% overall specificity. These results support the overall usefulness of the ASQ:SE to discriminate between children with social-emotional delays and those who appear to be developing typically in social-emotional areas.

To measure the utility of the ASQ:SE, parents ($N = 731$) completed utility questionnaires. More than 97% rated ASQ:SE items easy to understand and appropriate. Parents indicated that the ASQ:SE took little time to complete and helped them to think about social and emotional development in their young children.

3

Developing a Screening and Monitoring Program Using the ASQ:SE

ASQ:SE

This chapter presents detailed information on how to plan and develop a program designed to screen and monitor the social and emotional development of young children ages 3 to 66 months using the ASQ:SE. Planning of the program and collaboration with relevant community agencies prior to implementation is essential to the success of any relatively large-scale screening program that requires input and coordination across a variety of agencies and personnel. This chapter describes seven phases, beginning with initial planning and moving to implementation of a program designed to assist communities in the early identification of young children with potential social or emotional problems. Figure 3 shows these seven phases as linear. The development of a screening program may follow this linear sequence; however, program staff may have many valid reasons to address phases simultaneously or in a different sequence.

The purpose of screening and monitoring programs is twofold. One goal is to accurately identify children who should receive follow-up attention to determine if a problem exists. A second goal is to conduct the program in a manner that permits the assessment of large groups of children at low cost per child. Effective screening programs are able to acquire reliable targeted information on large groups of individuals in economical ways. Screening programs fail if the outcomes are in error (i.e., the information is inaccurate or unreliable) and if per individual costs are high (i.e., the cost of conducting the screening exceeds the usefulness of the outcome). Consequently, effective screening of children for social-emotional problems requires a tool or procedure that is low in cost to use and yields accurate outcomes (e.g., acceptable over- and underidentification rates).

Screening generally refers to a one-time administration of a tool or procedure. For example, kindergarten roundups are generally conducted as a one-time observation and testing of children before they enter first grade. Monitoring implies ongoing surveillance of the target population over time. For example, infants discharged from a neonatal intensive care

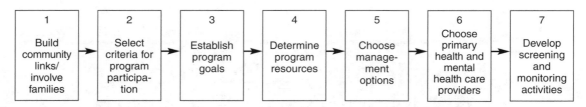

Figure 3.   Seven phases for developing a screening and monitoring program. These steps can be performed one at a time, or a few may be undertaken simultaneously. Sometimes program staff will choose to complete the steps in an order different from the one shown here.

unit might be tested at 6, 12, 24, and 36 months. The ASQ:SE can be used as a one-time screener, or, preferably, it can be used to monitor children over time by using the questionnaires at designated intervals. Consequently, the program described in this *User's Guide* is generally referred to as both a screening and monitoring program, although the terms are used separately.

PHASE 1: BUILD COMMUNITY LINKS/INVOLVE FAMILIES

One of the most important features of successful community mental health screening and intervention programs for young children is collaboration, or the establishment of connections between systems that historically have not interacted with one another (Knitzer, 2000). The pooling of knowledge and resources is particularly important when dealing with the complex issues surrounding young children's mental health. Because the roots of problems may or may not be organically based, issues such as the quality of parent–child interactions, drug and alcohol abuse, maternal depression, poverty, domestic violence, and child abuse should be dealt with concurrently for mental health interventions to have lasting effects.

A second important feature is to involve families in the planning and developing of the screening and monitoring program. Families' suggestions regarding procedures and agencies to include in the process generally provide a useful perspective.

Prior to implementation of a screening and monitoring program, links should be established among agencies whose expertise encompasses mental health, substance abuse, child protective services, social services, child care, education, special education, and public health. A useful place to begin is to arrange regular meetings or conversations with the Local Early Intervention Interagency Coordinating Council (LICC). The LICC is an interagency group that operates in most communities to coordinate services under IDEA 1997. The creation of work groups or the establishment of an ongoing dialogue among community agencies related to services for young children with social-emotional problems is essential to determining what services are currently available and where gaps exist.

Part C of IDEA 1997 establishes a program for the provision of intervention services to infants and toddlers and specifies the developmental services to be provided in the areas of physical, cognitive, communication, social-emotional, and adaptive development. Services included under Part C include family counseling, psychological services, social work services, occupational and physical therapy, speech therapy, and early identification through screening and assessment. These types of services should be available in every community for even the youngest child meeting state eligibility requirements. If services are not available, and the need is present, this service gap should be addressed by the LICC.

Part B of IDEA 1997 mandates special education and related services for children age 3 through 21. Section 619 of Part B pertains to children ages 3 through 5. Services included under Section 619 are education, occupational and physical therapy, speech therapy, and services for children with learning disabilities and with serious emotional disturbance. In most states, Section 619 services are provided by local school districts.

To begin establishing links between Part B and Part C services, the screening program can contact school districts and the lead agency for Part C services provision (which varies by state). Meetings can be arranged between these representatives and the screening program. In addition, mental health, Head Start, child protective services, and other human services and medical home visiting programs can be contacted. As previously mentioned, the LICC may have ongoing meetings with key agency personnel in attendance.

PHASE 2: SELECT CRITERIA FOR PROGRAM PARTICIPATION

Once community links between relevant agencies and personnel have been established, the next phase requires determining who should be the target of the screening and monitoring program. This phase often can and should be combined with Phase 3, establishing program goals. For many communities and agencies, selecting the target population is inseparable from selecting program goals.

Arriving at agreement about the general population to be screened and monitored may be straightforward. Most screening and monitoring programs are focused on children who are at risk; however, the number of children at risk in this country is very large and many communities do not have adequate resources to screen and monitor all children at risk over several years. Given large populations and limited resources, the development of objective criteria to define subgroups of the risk population to be screened is generally necessary.

A wide variety of risk factors affect individual children (Cicchetti & Toth, 2000; Duncan & Brooks-Gunn, 2000; Garbarino & Ganzel, 2000; Lyons-Ruth, Alpern, & Repacholi, 1993; Zeanah, 2000). These factors can potentially act as barriers to healthy social-emotional development. Studies that have monitored the development of risk populations over time report that the most reliable outcome predictors are not individual variables such as prematurity, teen parenthood, or poverty but rather the number of risk factors to which a child is exposed (Garbarino & Ganzel,

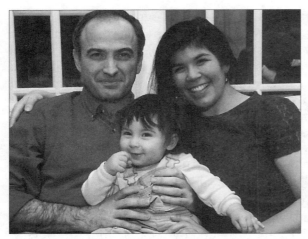

Photo by Terry Joseph Sam.

2000; Sameroff, 2000; Sameroff & Fiese, 2000; Sameroff, Seifer, Baldwin, & Baldwin, 1994). Children who experience two to three risk factors are far more likely to develop problems than children who are exposed to one risk factor. For children exposed to four or more risk factors, the likelihood of poor developmental outcomes is significantly increased. Such results strongly suggest that programs should use the number of risk factors as their primary criterion rather than select specific risk factors. Table 6 shows the number of risk factors and priority recommendations for screening and monitoring. It should be recognized, however, that there are a few risk factors—such as parental psychopathology—that often occur in conjunction with other risk factors such as substance abuse and child maltreatment and constitute severe dysfunction in parenting that can lead to serious maladjustment and behavior problems (Osofsky & Thompson, 2000; Rogosch, Cicchetti, Shields, & Toth, 1996). For example, maternal depression is known to contribute to maladaptive parenting and emotional problems in infants and children (Osofsky & Thompson, 2000; Weinberg & Tronick, 1997). Instances of parental psychopathology warrant careful monitoring of the child's social-emotional development.

Once the criteria are selected to determine the target population, they should be clearly written so that they are understood by personnel in community agencies who may refer or identify potentially eligible children/families. The selection criteria should also be formulated to be respectful of families to the greatest extent possible.

Table 6.   Recommended screening and monitoring priority for numbers of co-occurring risk factors

Number of co-occurring risk factors	Examples of risk factors	Screening and monitoring priority
Four or more	Poverty Abuse/neglect Substance abuse Teen parent	*Mandatory:* must be screened and monitored
Three	Parent mental illness Premature birth No high school education	*High:* should be screened and monitored if at all possible
Two	Chromosomal abnormality Abuse/neglect	*Moderate:* should be screened and monitored if resources allow
One	Parental substance abuse *or* poverty *or* teen parent	*Low:* screen and monitor if possible

PHASE 3: ESTABLISH PROGRAM GOALS

Before a screening and monitoring program is initiated, goals for the program should be established. Careful delineation of the program's goals and objectives by the major stakeholders (i.e., parents, program staff, community agency staff) will help to ensure that the program operates and uses resources efficiently and effectively. Several meetings of individuals from participating or receiving agencies may be required to develop a set of reasonable and generally acceptable goals. Time spent during this step is likely to result in a monitoring program that better meets child/family, community, regional, and state needs.

The following goals are offered as examples for monitoring programs designed to identify children with social-emotional problems:

- Increase understanding among families, care providers, and communities about the importance of nurturing healthy social-emotional development in young children.
- Conduct community-based screening of infants' and young children's social-emotional development at designated intervals.
- Identify infants and young children early and accurately who require further evaluation in the area of social-emotional competence.
- Increase involvement of parents in the assessment of their children's social-emotional health.
- Refer children for social-emotional evaluations and services when necessary in a timely manner.
- Identify professionals qualified to undertake comprehensive evaluation of young children's social-emotional development.
- Increase access to mental health–related services for infants, young children, and their families.

Program staff should modify these suggested goals to fit the needs of their community and screening program. After developing program goals, the next phase is to determine the resources available to operate the program and to allocate them appropriately.

PHASE 4: DETERMINE PROGRAM RESOURCES

The success of any monitoring program, no matter what its resources are, is dependent on matching its goals to available resources. For many programs, establishing goals and determining program resources are activities best done simultaneously. If these phases are conducted separately, it may be necessary to revise program goals once resources are analyzed and allocated.

Determining resources may require some modification of the chosen goals in at least three ways. First, limited resources may require changes in program goals. For example, a program may have set a goal to monitor

During training conducted at Green Waters Child Protective Services, personnel identified logistics and time constraints as potential barriers to screening and monitoring children in their foster care program. During the discussion, however, several participants were able to identify existing systems in the agency that could assist with screening efforts. For example, prior to every 6-month review of active cases, caseworkers would send a request for updated information to foster care providers. It was suggested that with this mailing, an ASQ:SE be enclosed for the foster parents to complete.

all infants discharged from the local hospital neonatal intensive care unit for a period of 3 years. An examination of resources may indicate that the necessary personnel and funds are not available to conduct such a large project. Resources may be available, however, to monitor a subgroup of infants who have three or more risk factors, thus requiring a modification in the program goal.

Second, modification of goals may also be necessary when a specific resource is not found to be available. Education-related resources may not be available for infants and toddlers (because of narrow IDEA 1997 eligibility definitions under Part C). Therefore, referral resources for families may be scarce, with community mental health services as the only resource available to a family until the child turns 3. In other instances,

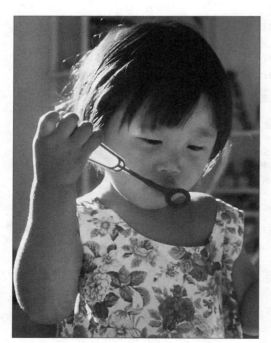

programs may have to narrow their focus. For example, a goal for a child protective services agency may be for caseworkers to screen and monitor children in foster care. Upon learning that the caseworkers are too busy to assume such a responsibility, the goal might be modified by shifting the assessment activities to personnel who are competent and able to take on the task.

Third, limited resources may require changes in the means by which a goal is accomplished. Conducting home visits to families of all children to be monitored may not be financially possible. The program may therefore choose to use a variety of methods for conducting monitoring, such as mailing questionnaires to parents who are able to complete them independently and reserving home visits for parents who require or desire assistance completing the questionnaires.

Table 7.   Options for using the ASQ:SE system

Administrator	Settings	Method of completion	Frequency of use	Method of distribution
Parent/guardian Mother Father Both parents Foster parents **Care provider** Child care provider Teacher/early interventionist **Both parent and care provider**	**Home** **Clinic** Primary health care clinics Immunization clinics Mental health clinics **Center based** Child care Preschool Baby groups **Other** Health fairs School screenings Community child-find activities	**Independent** **With assistance** Interview Translation	**One-time screening** **Ongoing monitoring** All ASQ:SE intervals Several ASQ:SE intervals	**Through mail** **At centers** **During home visits**

PHASE 5: CHOOSE MANAGEMENT OPTIONS

Program staff have a number of options when deciding how to use the ASQ:SE system. The following three factors are likely to affect the method chosen: 1) type of program, 2) available resources, and 3) characteristics of parents (e.g., cultural group, parent reading ability). Table 7 provides examples of options for programs implementing the ASQ:SE system.

Four Corners Head Start staff were interested in implementing a system to screen and monitor the social-emotional behaviors of the children in their Early Head Start program. The staff were concerned, however, about their ability to take on this task and follow up with children who were identified with possible problems. At the time, there was only one half-time child mental health specialist for an organization that served 500 families. The staff developed a two-level system in which ASQ:SE questionnaires were distributed by the teacher or home visitor to all families in the fall. The mental health specialist then limited her follow-up to families who did not return questionnaires and to children whose scores on the ASQ:SE indicated a potential problem. She contacted each of the 106 families who did not return questionnaires, by telephone or in person, and assisted them, when appropriate, in completing the ASQ:SE. For children with potential problems, she met with families individually and ascertained needs and assisted the families with gaining access to community resources.

As shown in Table 7, program staff have a number of options available for using the ASQ:SE, including how, where, and how often the questionnaires will be administered. Specific questions should address

1. Who should complete the ASQ:SE?
2. In what setting(s) will the ASQ:SE be used?
3. What method(s) of completion will be used?
4. How frequently will the ASQ:SE be used?
5. What method(s) of distribution will be used?

Each of these questions is addressed in the following sections.

Who Should Complete the ASQ:SE?

Parents, guardians, child care providers, and preschool teachers can complete an ASQ:SE on a child. It may be helpful when gathering information to have more than one person complete a questionnaire about each child because a child's behavior may vary greatly from setting to setting and behaviors that are problematic to one parent or care provider may not be of concern to another.

Parent/Guardian   The original ASQ and the ASQ:SE systems were both developed as parent-completed screening tools, and, in general, having parents complete the tool is the preferred method of use. There are many compelling reasons to include parents in the screening process, including the knowledge parents have about their children, the importance of understanding a parent's perspective, and the ability to respond to parent concerns. A significant need exists for program staff to identify parent concerns and respond to these concerns in a timely and supportive manner. It is also helpful, especially while assessing social-emotional development, to gather perspectives from both parents. What may be an urgent concern for one parent may be of little concern to the other.

Myrna Jo and her husband Bob brought Timmy, their 5-month-old, to a local feeding clinic. The young mother discussed the heartache she felt during mealtimes with Timmy, who was being fed through a gastrointestinal tube. However, in answering the ASQ:SE, Bob said that mealtimes with Timmy were enjoyable most of the time. Bob appeared not to experience the same stress that Myrna Jo was feeling. As they discussed the feeding question on the ASQ:SE ("Do you and your child enjoy mealtimes together?"), Myrna Jo was able to see Bob's perspective and why he thought Timmy was happy. Bob was also able to understand Myrna Jo's fear and anxiety at feeding times.

Care Provider and Teacher/Early Interventionist   Because many children spend a great deal of time in child care outside the home, it may be important to gather information from child care providers, teachers, and early interventionists as well as parents. Professional caregivers can complete the ASQ:SE; however, it is important that caregivers have 15–20 hours per week of contact with the child before completing an ASQ:SE. If caregivers complete the ASQ:SE in lieu of parents, every effort should be made to include parents in the screening process and to share information with them.

Both Parent and Care Provider   Some programs such as child care centers may choose to have both the parent and a child care worker complete the ASQ:SE independently and may then compare questionnaires. This method provides an excellent strategy to facilitate communication between a parent and a care provider about a child's behavior. Because a child's behaviors often differ across settings, there may be a discrepancy in ASQ:SE scores. Through discussion of these differences, valuable information about the child may surface.

Andrew is a 4-year-old child who was removed from his mother's home due to neglect. He has been in foster care for 6 months and was recently screened using the ASQ and the ASQ:SE. Because Andrew's mother currently has visitation rights with him for only 1 hour once a week, Andrew's foster mother was asked to complete the screening questionnaire. The caseworker chose to share results from the screening with Andrew's mother so that she could be kept informed of Andrew's overall developmental status.

In What Setting(s) Will the ASQ:SE Be Used?

The settings in which the ASQ:SE may be used include the home as well as clinical, center-based, and other settings that provide services to families with young children.

Home Settings   The ASQ:SE questionnaires were developed to be completed by parents at home or during a home visit. A home visit may be required when parents are unable to read, have other difficulties with independent completion of the questionnaires, or are unwilling or unable to travel to a center. Detailed information on the use of the ASQ:SE during a home visit can be found in Appendix B. The questionnaires may be a part of a larger home-visiting curriculum, for example, as part of an abuse and neglect prevention program. If used in a mail-out system, care must be taken to follow up on parents' noted concerns with a telephone call or home visit.

Clinical Settings   ASQ:SE questionnaires can be used by primary health care providers to gather screening information on a child prior to a physical examination. Health care providers may save time by sending questionnaires to parents prior to their appointments or by having parents complete the questionnaire while waiting for their appointments. This method helps parents identify concerns prior to their appointment and provides a focus for the examination and subsequent discussion.

Center-Based Settings   The ASQ:SE may be used in child care and educational settings. In addition to using the tool for screening purposes, use of the ASQ:SE in this type of setting may help to facilitate discussion between teachers and parents about a child's behavior across settings. As mentioned previously, if someone other than a parent completes the ASQ:SE, he or she should have at least 15–20 hours per week of contact with the child.

Other Settings   The ASQ:SE can be used in other programs whose purpose is finding children in need of special services, monitoring a child's development, or educating parents about the development of their young children. Examples of other settings include health fairs sponsored by Head Start programs, kindergarten round-ups offered by school districts, and child-find screenings conducted by early intervention programs.

What Method(s) of Completion Will Be Used?

The ASQ:SE can be completed by parents independently or with assistance as needed. When interviewers or translators are assisting with administering the ASQ:SE, they should be careful to clarify their role, which is to read items and gather information from the parent. The ASQ:SE has some items that may be considered subjective by parents. For example, the question, "Does your child scream, cry, or have tantrums for long periods of time?" may cause a parent to inquire about what might be considered a long period. To the extent possible, the interviewer should not advise or lead parents but should encourage parents to use their judgment in answering questionnaire items.

Independent   The ASQ:SE was designed to be completed by most parents independently, which accounts for its low cost per child served. Questionnaires can be given to parents or mailed to them for completion. When using the questionnaires in these ways, it is important to monitor their timely return.

With Assistance   Program staff should be prepared to offer assistance to parents who request or need it during questionnaire completion.

Interview   The ASQ:SE can be completed through an interview over the telephone or in person. Using the ASQ:SE as an interview tool may be appropriate for parents with limited reading skills or poor understanding of written questions as a result of language, cognitive, or mental health difficulties. Suggestions for conducting interviews can be found in Appendix B.

Translation   The ASQ:SE system can be used to screen children using the services of a translator over the telephone or during face-to-face contact. Translating the ASQ:SE may be necessary for parents who are not fluent in English or Spanish. When using this method, it is necessary for the translator(s) to carefully review all items and come to an agreement with the administering program as to the intent of the items and what would be an appropriate translation. Because research on the ASQ:SE has only been conducted on the English and Spanish versions of the tool, results of questionnaires that are administered in other languages should be viewed with caution.

How Frequently Will the ASQ:SE Be Used?

The ASQ:SE can be used to screen a child's social-emotional development at one point in time or may be used to monitor a child repeatedly using more than one ASQ:SE interval.

One-Time Screening   Although the ASQ:SE system was developed to monitor children over time, the questionnaires can be also used for one-time screening. Some programs may not be able to mount a full-time monitoring program but be able to screen children once. For example, programs that work with homeless individuals may encounter situations in which only a one-time screening is possible. Programs that choose this approach should be prepared to respond immediately to concerns that parents note or to make a referral if appropriate. For example, programs should have information on hand about a variety of topics (e.g., toilet training, feeding) or should have staff members who can discuss these concerns with the parents. Staff should be prepared to refer children for follow-up when it is indicated by screening results and conversations with the parents.

Ongoing Monitoring   Repeatedly screening children over time is referred to as *monitoring*. The extent of monitoring (e.g., number of children, number of age intervals) is highly dependent on program resources. Programs with substantial resources may use all of the available ASQ:SE intervals (i.e., 6, 12, 18, 24, 30, 36, 48, and 60 months). Programs with fewer resources may choose specific intervals for their monitoring efforts. Considering the rapid development and change that occurs in children between the ages of birth and 5 years, it is advisable to monitor children's development over time. Any change in children's homes, schools, or health status may greatly affect the status of their social-emotional development.

What Method(s) of Distribution Will Be Used?

The ASQ:SE questionnaires can be distributed to parents in at least three different ways, including through the mail, at centers, and during home visit.

Through the Mail   The ASQ:SE questionnaires were primarily designed to be completed by parents at home. In comparison to the cost of approaches that employ highly skilled professionals, the cost of using the mail-out system is extremely modest (Chan & Taylor, 1998). See Appendix B for specific steps designed for the use and tracking of questionnaires when using a mail-out system.

A common concern about using the questionnaires in the mail-out format is the return rate. Many screening programs use the questionnaires in this format, and a variety of ideas for increasing return rates has been generated. Following are ideas that program staff have found successful in increasing return rates:

- Provide a self-addressed, stamped envelope with the questionnaire
- Call parents after the questionnaire has been mailed to them and after it is returned to provide feedback on screening results
- Provide incentives to return the questionnaire (e.g., food coupons, small gifts)
- Respond quickly and appropriately to parents' concerns
- Send an activity sheet (see Appendix C) or information related to parental concerns that were marked on the questionnaire (e.g., toileting tips, age-appropriate discipline ideas)

At Centers Physicians' offices, health clinics, and community-based programs can distribute the ASQ:SE to parents. For example, when parents bring their child in for a well check-up, they can be asked to complete a questionnaire. Or, early intervention programs may ask parents to complete questionnaires on an annual basis.

During Home Visits During home visits, parents can be given a questionnaire and asked to complete it, or the questionnaire can be completed through an interview.

PHASE 6: INVOLVE PRIMARY HEALTH AND MENTAL HEALTH CARE PROVIDERS

Primary health and mental health care providers in most communities wish to be kept informed about their young patients' participation in screening and monitoring programs. Primary health care providers may conduct a developmental assessment of their patients or may want to be notified if such an assessment is conducted by another community agency. Figure 4 contains a sample letter to a primary health care provider from program staff explaining the family's participation in the monitoring program.

Staff who are conducting screening and monitoring programs should involve primary health and mental health care providers of participating children for four important reasons. First, health care providers have valuable information about their patients and young children in general that may serve to enhance monitoring efforts. Second, collaboration among professionals and program personnel will produce the greatest benefits for young children and their families. Third, primary health care providers may have the ability to make the referrals that are necessary for further diagnostic assessments and/or services for young children and their families. Fourth, health care providers need to be aware of services being provided to their patients so that services are not duplicated.

PHASE 7: DEVELOP SCREENING AND MONITORING ACTIVITIES

The target areas and associated activities shown in Table 8 are necessary to operate most screening programs. Before a screening and monitoring program is implemented, it is important to outline staff responsibilities and determine how referrals will be made. Clear, well-delineated responsibilities for staff will allow for efficient systems to be created and maintained over time. Training related to these job responsibilities is a key factor in creating systems that work for staff and families.

SUMMARY

Time devoted to the planning steps described in this chapter is well spent in terms of ensuring the long-term success of a screening and monitoring program. The seven phases for developing this kind of program provide a foundation for the day-to-day activities of using the ASQ:SE system with young children and their families. In the next chapter, the use of the ASQ:SE is described in detail, including keeping track of the question-

---

Dear Dr. [fill in physician's name]:

The parents or guardian of your patient [fill in child's name] have agreed to participate in a monitoring program. The purpose of this project is to provide follow-along screening to infants and children who are at risk for developmental problems. Parents or guardians are asked to respond to questions about their child's social and emotional development at repeated intervals from approximately 6 months to 5 years. If a child obtains a score above an established cutoff point on a questionnaire, the parent or guardian and physician are notified so that further evaluation can be scheduled.

If you would like more information about the project, please contact [fill in staff member's name and telephone number].

Sincerely,

[fill in staff member's name]
[fill in program name]

The ASQ:SE User's Guide, Squires, Bricker, and Twombly. © 2002 Paul H. Brookes Publishing Co.

Figure 4.   Sample letter from a program staff member explaining the screening and monitoring program to a physician.

Table 8.   Target areas and associated activities necessary to operate an ASQ:SE screening and monitoring program

Target area	Activities
Questionnaire management	Activities related to keeping track of child and family information, questionnaires, and questionnaire activities. See Chapter 4 and Appendix B for more information about this process.
Questionnaire completion	Activities related to getting questionnaires to parents for completion and providing whatever level of assistance is necessary to support a parent's ability to complete the questionnaires.
Questionnaire scoring and interpretation of results	Activities related to scoring, interpreting, and decision making based on ASQ:SE results. At this level, it is important to create a system to help support staff with follow-up decisions. Creating job responsibilities in which supervisors or mental health specialists are available to discuss ASQ:SE results or to help problem solve concerns is critical to a system that is supportive of staff and, ultimately, families.
Follow-up and referral	Activities related to follow-up and referral services based on ASQ:SE results. It is important to determine who is responsible for follow-up services and what timelines are acceptable.
Evaluation	Activities related to evaluation of screening systems. Systems should be evaluated periodically by staff and families to determine what is working and what could be done differently to improve on the process.

naires, preparing the master set of the ASQ:SE, introducing the screening program to parents, administering and scoring the questionnaires, and interpreting results. Forms to assist with organizing and maintaining the monitoring system are included.

4

Using the ASQ:SE System

ASQ:SE

Once program personnel have completed the seven planning and development phases described in Chapter 3, they are ready to use the ASQ:SE system to screen and monitor the target population of children. This chapter discusses how the questionnaire system functions and has been organized around the following activities:

1. Keeping track of the questionnaires
2. Preparing the master set of the ASQ:SE
3. Introducing the screening program to parents
4. Completing the questionnaires
5. Scoring the questionnaires
6. Interpreting ASQ:SE results

PHASE 1: KEEP TRACK OF THE QUESTIONNAIRES

When monitoring large numbers of children over time, it is essential that accurate and efficient procedures be adopted to permit timely distribution and completion of questionnaires. The integrity of the ASQ:SE system is dependent upon reasonable adherence to a preset schedule. The schedule ensures that parents or service providers receive and complete questionnaires in a timely manner, within 3 months on either side of younger age intervals (i.e., the 6, 12, 18, 24, and 30 month intervals) and 6 months on either side of the older age intervals (i.e., the 36, 48, and 60 month intervals). Table 9 provides guidelines for which interval is appropriate for a child's age. The ASQ:SE questionnaires, unlike the ASQ questionnaires, do not correct for prematurity. This is because of the larger time frame covered by each ASQ:SE interval and the less significant relationship between social-emotional development and prematurity. If programs are monitoring the child using the ASQ and have assigned a corrected date of birth (CDOB), personnel may use the CDOB for the ASQ:SE questionnaires as well. (The CDOB is often used until the child

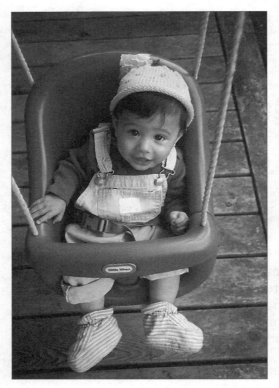

is 24 months of age, at which time the actual date of birth should be used.) Appendix B contains detailed information on how to assemble a child's file, including forms that programs may use.

Questionnaire Management Systems

Timely questionnaire distribution and receipt can be accomplished by 1) developing your own system, 2) using a card file, or 3) using a computer-based tickler system. Individuals who monitor relatively small groups of children often develop their own systems to keep track of questionnaire activities, for example, entering target dates (for questionnaire completion) in their individual day planners. A system used to monitor large groups of children (e.g., a few hundred) is a card file tickler system. The card file has been used successfully by many programs that use the ASQ system. One staff person is appointed to manage the card files and either mails the questionnaires or makes direct service providers aware of which children require screening activities. Appendix B contains instructions for the use of a card file tickler system that is adaptable to a mail-back system and other uses of the questionnaires. Computer systems rely on database software that is modified to fit individual program needs. Systems for more than several hundred children (e.g., statewide programs) generally need to use a computer-based system to keep track of the questionnaires. Another strategy program staff have found useful is to attach a notice to a child's file to complete a screening during other ongoing activities (e.g. immunizations, well-baby checkups, 6-month case reviews).

Table 9.   ASQ:SE interval completion guidelines

If child's age is between:	Use this ASQ:SE interval:
3 months, 0 days, and 8 months, 29 days	6 month
9 months, 0 days, and 14 months, 29 days	12 month
15 months, 0 days, and 20 months, 29 days	18 month
21 months, 0 days, and 26 months, 29 days	24 month
27 months, 0 days, and 32 months, 29 days	30 month
33 months, 0 days, and 41 months, 29 days	36 month
42 months, 0 days, and 53 months, 29 days	48 month
54 months, 0 days, and 65 months, 29 days	60 month

PHASE 2: PREPARE THE MASTER SET OF THE ASQ:SE

The ASQ:SE questionnaires are designed to be photocopied as needed by program staff.[1] Each age interval's master questionnaire features a different color for easy recognition by the staff in charge of photocopying and/ or distributing the questionnaires. The method of use selected by the program or agency will affect the way in which questionnaires are distributed and used; however, some general guidelines do apply to all users. The first page of each questionnaire provides a space for programs to stamp, type, or write essential program identifying information to individualize protocols prior to copying. Some programs may choose to affix or stamp a logo as well. Figure 5 presents an example for Steps-Ahead, a program that screens and monitors children at risk for developmental and social-emotional delay. Identifying information is vital when mail-out procedures are used. The name of a contact person may also be indicated to give parents access to a resource person who can answer questions or address concerns. The first page of the questionnaire also contains a summary of important points for parents to remember. This list provides a space for staff to indicate when the questionnaire should be completed and a contact name and telephone number in case the parent has any questions.

In each boxed master set of questionnaires, a master mail-out and mail-back form is provided. For programs that decide to use a mail-out format, the name of the screening program and its address should be stamped, printed, or typed on the mail-back portion (bottom) of the page, and the parent's name and address should be written or typed on the mail-out portion (top) of the page. Staff may prefer to use an envelope to mail the questionnaires; in these cases, a stamped return envelope should also be enclosed to encourage return of the completed questionnaires. Detailed information on the use of mailing the ASQ:SE can be found in Appendix B. In addition, an example of a mail-back and mail-out master form can be found in Figure B6 in Appendix B.

---

[1]*Purchasers of the **Ages & Stages Questionnaires: Social-Emotional (ASQ:SE): A Parent-Completed, Child-Monitoring System for Social-Emotional Behaviors** are granted permission to photocopy the questionnaires as well as the sample letters and forms in **The ASQ:SE User's Guide for the Ages & Stages Questionnaires: Social-Emotional: A Parent-Completed, Child-Monitoring System for Social-Emotional Behaviors** in the course of their agency's service provision to families.* Each branch office that will be using the ASQ:SE system must purchase its own set of original questionnaires; master forms cannot be shared among sites. The questionnaires and samples are meant to be used to facilitate screening and monitoring and to assist in the early identification of children who may need further evaluation. Electronic reproduction of the questionnaires is prohibited, and none of the ASQ:SE materials may be reproduced to generate revenue for any program or individual. Photocopies may only be made from an original set of color-coded master questionnaires and/or an original **User's Guide.** Programs are prohibited from charging parents, caregivers, or other service providers who will be completing and/or scoring the questionnaires fees in excess of the exact cost to photocopy the master forms. Likewise, the ASQ:SE materials may not be used in a way contrary to the family-oriented philosophies of the ASQ:SE developers. *Unauthorized use beyond this privilege is prosecutable under federal law.* You will see the copyright protection line at the bottom of each form.

For other questions pertaining to the ASQ:SE, please contact the Rights Department, Paul H. Brookes Publishing Co., Post Office Box 10624, Baltimore, MD 21285-0624, USA; 1-410-337-9580.

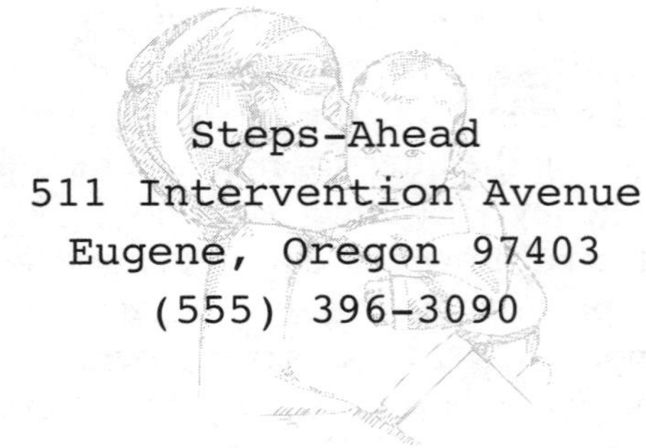

Steps–Ahead
511 Intervention Avenue
Eugene, Oregon 97403
(555) 396–3090

Figure 5.   On the first page of each questionnaire, important program identifying information should be added. In this example, the staff at Steps-Ahead have entered the program's name, address, and telephone number for the easy reference of parents and service providers.

PHASE 3: INTRODUCE THE SCREENING PROGRAM TO PARENTS

Ideally, the initial introduction of a family to the ASQ:SE system will be done by a program staff member. While some programs may not have the resources necessary to visit each family, every effort should be made to make this process as user friendly and personal as possible. If program staff cannot visit the home, a telephone conversation should be scheduled. While introducing the ASQ:SE, it is critical to set a positive tone and establish open communication with a family member. The tone and sensitivity of this initial introduction may encourage or deter a parent's participation in the program. Be clear about the purpose of the screening program, about who will have access to screening information, and about how the screening results will be used. For example, family members involved with child protective services may be concerned about how their answers will be interpreted. If parents admit that their child is out of control or has hurt other children, they may be concerned about how this information will be used and who will have access to it. A letter such as the one found in Figure 6 can be attached to the first ASQ:SE questionnaire to remind parents of the purpose of the monitoring program. The letter contains a brief description of the importance of early development, a description of the monitoring program, an explanation of the amount of parent participation expected, and a description of the program's activities.

Obtain Consent

Obtaining written consent from a child's parent or guardian should be a prerequisite for participation in the program. It is important to provide parents with adequate information about the screening and monitoring program when obtaining their consent to participate. Figure 7 is an ex-

---

ASQ☺SE

Dear [fill in parents' or guardians' names]:

The first 5 years of life are very important to your child because this time sets the stage for success in school and later life. During infancy and early childhood, many experiences should be gained and many skills learned. It is important to ensure that each child's development is proceeding without problem during this period; therefore, we are interested in helping you follow your child's social and emotional development. You can help us by completing a questionnaire that will be mailed to you at 6- to 12-month intervals. You will be asked to answer questions about some things your child does and does not do and to mail the questionnaire back to [fill in staff member's name].

If the completed questionnaire indicates that your child seems to be developing without problems, we will send a letter stating that your child's social and emotional development appears to be progressing well. We will mail the next age-level questionnaire to you at the appropriate time.

If you have concerns about your baby at any time, you can reach a staff person at any time to discuss your concerns. If the completed questionnaire suggests that there are concerns about your child, we will contact you directly, and you may wish to have your child's doctor or another agency conduct a further examination. All information about your child and your family will be kept confidential.

Sincerely,

[fill in staff member's name]
[fill in program name]

The ASQ:SE User's Guide, Squires, Bricker, and Twombly. © 2002 Paul H. Brookes Publishing Co.

Figure 6.   Sample information and agreement letter to parents or guardians. This letter should be modified by personnel to reflect the ASQ:SE method(s) to be used by the program. A Spanish translation of this letter is provided in Appendix G.

ample of a consent form for parents or guardians to indicate their willingness or refusal to participate in the screening and monitoring program. This form should accompany the introductory letter, such as the one shown in Figure 6. Parents' willingness to be (and remain) involved in the program may hinge on understanding expectations for their involvement. This consent form should be modified as necessary to meet the specific needs of a program. If appropriate, this is a good point at which to ask parents whether they would like assistance completing the questionnaires.

Some program personnel have found that it is easier to obtain parental consent by simply presenting the screening and monitoring process as part of the overall services that are offered in their program. For example, a statewide child care program in Florida assists low-income families with their child care costs. When a family enrolls in the subsidized child care program, the screening and monitoring program is sometimes presented as one of the additional services that families receive. When families sign their consent to participate in the subsidized child care program, they are agreeing to participate in the screening and monitoring program. If a family does not want to have their child screened, they must sign a separate "refusal to participate" form.

ASQ:SE

______ I have read the description of the monitoring program, and I wish to participate. I am willing to fill out questionnaires about my child's development and mail them back promptly.

______ I have read the description of the monitoring project. I understand the purpose of this project and do not wish to participate.

Parent's or guardian's signature ______________________

Date ______________

Child's name ______________________

Child's birthdate ______________

Child's primary physician ______________________

Figure 7. Sample of a participation agreement to be signed by a child's parent or guardian before beginning implementation procedures. A Spanish translation of this form is provided in Appendix G.

Collect Demographic Information

After parents or guardians have signed a form indicating their willingness to participate in the program, parents can be asked to provide demographic information about their child and family. Ideally, this information is obtained in person, but it can also be gathered over the telephone or through the mail. A sample demographic form on which to record this information can be found in Figure B1 in Appendix B.

PHASE 4: COMPLETE THE QUESTIONNAIRES

Prior to completing the ASQ:SE, program staff need to determine how the questionnaire will be distributed (e.g., mail-out, interview). (Step-by-step guidance related to using the ASQ:SE in a mail-out or interview format or during a home visit is included in Appendix B.) In addition, the screening and monitoring program will need to be explained to parents and their consent to participate obtained. The next step is to assist parents in becoming familiar with the questionnaires, to review for parents the purpose of the ASQ:SE, and to explain how the information will be used. When introducing the questionnaires to parents, be sure to address the following:

1. Discuss the purpose of the ASQ:SE to parents and how the information gathered will be used.

   - The purpose of the ASQ:SE is to gain information on children's social and emotional development and parents' feelings about their child's development. Following is an example of language that program staff could use while introducing the ASQ:SE to parents:

*"This questionnaire asks about your child's social-emotional be-
haviors. Some of the questions are not very specific, but you
should answer based on your feelings or opinions about your
child's behavior."*

- It is important that parents understand how information gathered
from the ASQ:SE will be used. Some parents may have concerns
about confidentiality issues or may worry that information will
be used against them. Establishing trust between program staff
and parents is an important first step to gathering reliable information. This may be a difficult path for program staff to walk,
given mandatory reporting laws on child abuse and neglect, but is
a concern that needs to be addressed and discussed with parents.
Depending on the administering program, information gathered
may be used to 1) make a referral for diagnostic evaluation, 2) help
monitor the child's social-emotional development, and 3) help determine information or support services that families may need.
Program staff could say to parents: *"The information on this questionnaire will remain confidential. I will not be sharing the information with anyone without your consent. Your answers will
help me know what type of information I may be able to gather
for you. If you have questions or concerns about any of your
child's behaviors that are not within my expertise, there may be
other agencies in our community that can help."*

2. Discuss scoring options. With the exception of the open-ended questions at the end of each ASQ:SE questionnaire, each question has
three possible answer responses, which should be checked as appropriate:

- *Most of the time,* indicating the child is doing the behavior most
of the time, too much, or too often
- *Sometimes,* indicating the child is doing the behavior occasionally but not consistently
- *Rarely or never,* indicating the child rarely performs the behavior
or has never performed the behavior

Program staff should discuss these response options with parents before the parents complete the ASQ:SE, but staff should not provide
their opinions about how to answer the questionnaire. If a parent asks
for assistance to understand or interpret items, staff should try to reflect the question back to the parent and encourage the parent to provide his or her "best answer." Staff should try to provide as little interpretation about questions as possible, other than to help the parent
understand what is being asked by the item.

Note: It is important to emphasize that the *rarely or never* scoring option does allow for a child to have performed a behavior that is

Please read each question carefully and 1. Check the box ❑ that best describes your child's behavior *and* 2. Check the circle ❍ if this behavior is a concern	MOST OF THE TIME	SOMETIMES	RARELY OR NEVER	CHECK IF THIS IS A CONCERN
1. When upset, can your baby calm down within a half hour?	☑ z	❑ v	❑ x	❍
2. Does your baby smile at you and other family members?	❑ z	☑ v	❑ x	❍
3. Does your baby like to be picked up and held?	❑ z	❑ v	☑ x	✓

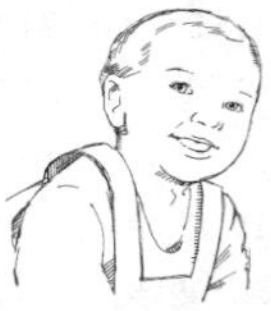

Figure 8. ASQ:SE scoring options for behaviors and concerns.

only a rare occurrence. For example, a child may become very clingy when ill but otherwise may be quite independent and outgoing. This clinging behavior is not part of the child's typical repertoire. The *sometimes* option refers to behaviors that are part of a child's repertoire, and may be of slight (or considerable) concern to a parent. On occasion parents overuse the *sometimes* response, resulting in an inflated score on the ASQ:SE.

3. Discuss how to mark concerns and open-ended questions. The circle in the far right column next to each question should be checked if the behavior is of concern to the parents. Sometimes parents check only the concern column but fail to check one of the scoring options. Encourage parents to check a scoring response first and then indicate if the behavior is of concern (see Figure 8). At the end of each questionnaire are two to three open-ended questions that ask about overall parental concerns; concerns related to the child's eating, sleeping, and toileting behaviors; and what parents enjoy most about their child. Parents should be encouraged to respond to these questions as appropriate.

PHASE 5: SCORE THE QUESTIONNAIRES

The questionnaires contain between 19 and 33 scored questions related to a child's behavior and an additional set of general unscored questions about eating, sleeping, and toileting concerns; overall worries about the child; and what parents enjoy about their child. General scoring guidelines are contained in Figure 9. Information related to scoring questionnaires with items left unanswered and interpreting parents' comments is

6 Month ASQ:SE Information Summary

Child's name: _____   Child's date of birth: _____

Person filling out the ASQ:SE: _____   Relationship to child: _____

Mailing address: _____   City: _____ State: _____ ZIP: _____

Telephone: _____   Assisting in ASQ:SE completion: _____

Today's date: _____   Administering program/provider: _____

SCORING GUIDELINES

1. Make sure the parent has answered all questions and has checked the concern column as necessary. If all questions have been answered, go to Step 2. If not all questions have been answered, you should first try to contact the parent to obtain answers or, if necessary, calculate an average score (see pages 39 and 41 of *The ASQ:SE User's Guide*).

2. Review any parent comments. If there are no comments, go to Step 3. If a parent has written in a response, see the section titled "Parent Comments" on pages 39, 41, and 42 of *The ASQ:SE User's Guide* to determine if the response indicates a behavior that may be of concern.

3. Using the following point system:

Z (for zero) next to the checked box	= 0 points
V (for Roman numeral V) next to the checked box	= 5 points
X (for Roman numeral X) next to the checked box	= 10 points
Checked concern	= 5 points

Add together:

Total points on page 3	= _____
Total points on page 4	= _____
Total points on page 5	= _____
Child's total score =	_____

SCORE INTERPRETATION

1. *Review questionnaires*

    Review the parent's answers to questions. Give special consideration to any individual questions that score 10 or 15 points and any written or verbal comments that the parent shares. Offer guidance, support, and information to families, and refer if necessary, as indicated by score and referral considerations.

2. *Transfer child's total score*

    In the table below, enter the child's total score (transfer total score from above).

Questionnaire interval	Cutoff score	Child's ASQ:SE score
6 months	45	

3. *Referral criteria*

    Compare the child's total score with the cutoff in the table above. If the child's score falls above the cutoff and the factors in Step 4 have been considered, refer the child for a mental health evaluation.

4. *Referral considerations*

    It is always important to look at assessment information in the context of other factors influencing a child's life. Consider the following variables prior to making referrals for a mental health evaluation. Refer to pages 44–46 in *The ASQ:SE User's Guide* for additional guidance related to these factors and for suggestions for follow-up.

    *   Setting/time factors
        (e.g., Is the child's behavior the same at home as at school? Have there been any stressful events in the child's life recently?)

    *   Development factors
        (e.g., Is the child's behavior related to a developmental stage or a developmental delay?)

    *   Health factors
        (e.g., Is the child's behavior related to health or biological factors?)

    *   Family/cultural factors
        (e.g., Is the child's behavior acceptable given cultural or family context?)

6

ASQ:SE   **6 months**

Figure 9.   ASQ:SE Information Summary with steps for scoring and interpreting scores.

discussed. In addition, information on use of the ASQ:SE Information Summary is provided.

Scoring Questionnaires with Unanswered Items: Average Scores

If a parent does not provide answers to all of the items on a questionnaire, attempts should be made to contact the parent as soon as possible to obtain responses to missing items. If the missing responses are provided, the scorer should follow the steps outlined in Figure 9. Sometimes parents omit an item because they are unsure of how to respond or have a concern about their child's behavior. Occasionally parents may not respond to an item because it is culturally inappropriate or inappropriate for their family's values. For these reasons, it is important to attempt to reach parents when items are left unanswered. Answers to questions should be obtained whenever possible, assuming that those answers do not compromise a family's culture or value system.

When a parent cannot be contacted and no more than two questions on the 6 to 18 month intervals or three questions on the 24 to 60 month intervals are left unanswered, an average score may be calculated (see Figure 10). An average score is computed by dividing the questionnaire's total points (child's total score for answered items) by the number of items answered. This formula yields an average score between 0 and 10. The average score is then multiplied by the number of unanswered questions and added to the child's total score, giving a final total score, which is used to compare with the cutoff point on the ASQ:SE Information Summary. An example of calculating an average score is shown in Figure 11.

Parent Comments

Throughout the ASQ:SE there are questions that provide space for parent comments. The questions with space for comments are discussed next, along with some guidelines for interpreting parents' answers.

All Intervals: Eating Problems   On the 6 month questionnaire, the question "Does your baby have any eating problems such as gagging, vomiting, or _____?" provides a space for the parent to write in another problem their child may be experiencing (e.g., refuses solid foods). This question is modified in the older intervals as "Does your child have eating problems such as stuffing foods, vomiting, eating nonfood items, or _____?" This question is targeting severe eating difficulties such as eating *only* one food item or only one food texture. If parents write comments that seem within developmental norms (e.g., their child is a picky eater) and they have no concerns about the child's behavior, program staff have the choice to either follow up with the parent after a few weeks or to seek advice from a feeding or nutritional expert.

18 Months and Older: Perseverative Behaviors   The question "Does your child do things over and over and can't seem to stop? Exam-

---

1. Compute average score:

$$\frac{\text{total points of questionnaire}}{\text{(child's total score for items answered)}} = \text{average score}$$
$$\text{total number of items answered}$$

2. Compute final total score:

total points of questionnaire +
(average score × number of unanswered items) = final total score

---

Figure 10.   Formulas to calculate the final total score from an average score on the ASQ:SE.

ples are rocking, hand flapping, spinning, or _____?" is designed to identify stereotypic or perseverative behaviors. A parent may write in a behavior that is a favored activity of the child (e.g., reading books, singing songs, playing tea party), and that behavior may not be of concern to the parent. When interpreting responses to this item, staff may use their professional judgment as to whether the behavior is atypical or can ask the parent for more information. Questions may help distinguish a true perseverative behavior, such as "How difficult is it for your child to stop the behavior?" or "What happens when you try to stop your child from doing this behavior?"

All Intervals: Others' Concerns   The question "Has anyone expressed concerns about your baby's (child's) behavior?" appears as the last scored question on all intervals. This question provides a glimpse into others' perceptions of the child's behavior. In many cases, a child care

---

Example: On the 36 month ASQ:SE, there are a total of 31 scored items. A parent answered 28 of 31 questions. The parent checked 24 items with 0 points; 1 item with 10 points, 3 items with 5 points each, and 1 concern (5 points) and left 3 items blank. The child's total score (for answered items) for the questionnaire is 30 points (10 + 15 + 5). The average score (30 points ÷ 28 items) equals 1.07. This number is the "best-guess point value" for each of the missing items. Because there are three missing items, 1.07 is multiplied by 3 and then added to the child's total score. The final total score (30 + [1.07 × 3]) is 33.21 points.

Child's total score for items answered   **= 30 points**

Average score   = $\dfrac{30 \text{ (child's total score)}}{28 \text{ (number of items answered)}}$ **= 1.07 points**

Final total score = 30 (total score) + 1.07 (average score)
                              × 3 (number of items unanswered)   **= 33.21 points**

The cutoff for the 36 month ASQ:SE questionnaire is **59 points;** therefore this score is below the cutoff point. A child with this score would be considered within the typical range. The monitoring program will ask the parent to complete the 48 month ASQ:SE in 6–12 months to continue monitoring the child's social and emotional status. Rather than use the average score, however, it is preferable to contact the parent to obtain the answers to unmarked questions or to find out why the parent did not complete the specific items.

Figure 11.   Example of calculating an average score and a final total score on the ASQ:SE.

provider or a relative may have commented on a child's behavior, even though a parent may not feel any concerns. This item provides an opportunity for parents to describe the comments of friends and relatives concerning their child's behavior.

All Intervals: Open-Ended Questions (Unscored)   Every interval includes an unscored, open-ended item asking whether the parent has concerns about the child's eating and sleeping behaviors. On the 30, 36, 48, and 60 month intervals, this question also asks whether the parent has concerns about the child's toilet training or toileting behaviors. An overall question, "Is there anything that worries you about your baby (child)?" is included on each interval. These open-ended questions are not scored but should serve as general indicators of parental concerns. Program staff should respond to any concerns noted in this section. A referral may be made based solely on a parent's response to an open-ended question, even if a child's ASQ:SE scores fall within a typical range.

In addition, each interval asks what the parent enjoys most about the child. This final question lets the parent finish the questionnaire on a positive note.

ASQ:SE Information Summary

The final two pages of each questionnaire make up the ASQ:SE Information Summary. The ASQ:SE Information Summary contains the same information across all age intervals, including identifying information about the child and family, instructions for scoring the questionnaire, a chart indicating cutoff scores for referrals, and a list of considerations that interventionists should be aware of prior to making referrals to mental health professionals. An example of a completed ASQ:SE Information Summary is shown in Figure 12.

This form was designed to be used by program staff to summarize assessment information and to help with the decision-making process. Some of the sections of this form would be unclear and therefore inappropriate for parents to complete by themselves. The ASQ:SE Information Summary should not be sent to a family if programs are using a mail-out method to administer the questionnaires. It is recommended that the form be completed by program staff to score questionnaires and review cutoffs and used in a guided interview format with parents for gathering information related to the Referral Considerations listed on the form.

PHASE 6: INTERPRET ASQ:SE RESULTS

After totaling the items and considering parent comments, a decision related to referral or follow-up preventive interventions will need to be made.

30 Month ASQ:SE Information Summary

Child's name: _Caleb Smith_   Child's date of birth: _3-8-99_

Person filling out the ASQ:SE: _Mary Smith_   Relationship to child: _Mother_

Mailing address: _42 Heathcliff Terrace_   City: _Seattle_   State: _WA_   ZIP: _98110_

Telephone: _555-7327_   Assisting in ASQ:SE completion: _____

Today's date: _9-18-01_   Administering program/provider: _Sandy Point El Svcs._

SCORING GUIDELINES

1. Make sure the parent has answered all questions and has checked the concern column as necessary. If all questions have been answered, go to Step 2. If not all questions have been answered, you should first try to contact the parent to obtain answers or, if necessary, calculate an average score (see pages 39 and 41 of *The ASQ:SE User's Guide*).

2. Review any parent comments. If there are no comments, go to Step 3. If a parent has written in a response, see the section titled "Parent Comments" on pages 39, 41, and 42 of *The ASQ:SE User's Guide* to determine if the response indicates a behavior that may be of concern.

3. Using the following point system:

Z (for zero) next to the checked box	= 0 points
V (for Roman numeral V) next to the checked box	= 5 points
X (for Roman numeral X) next to the checked box	= 10 points
Checked concern	= 5 points

   Add together:

Total points on page 3	= _40_
Total points on page 4	= _30_
Total points on page 5	= _0_
Total points on page 6	= _0_
Child's total score =	_70_

SCORE INTERPRETATION

1. *Review questionnaires*

   Review the parent's answers to questions. Give special consideration to any individual questions that score 10 or 15 points and any written or verbal comments that the parent shares. Offer guidance, support, and information to families, and refer if necessary, as indicated by score and referral considerations.

2. *Transfer child's total score*

   In the table below, enter the child's total score (transfer total score from above).

Questionnaire interval	Cutoff score	Child's ASQ:SE score
30 months	57	_70_

3. *Referral criteria*

   Compare the child's total score with the cutoff in the table above. If the child's score falls above the cutoff and the factors in Step 4 have been considered, refer the child for a mental health evaluation.

4. *Referral considerations*

   It is always important to look at assessment information in the context of other factors influencing a child's life. Consider the following variables prior to making referrals for a mental health evaluation. Refer to pages 44–46 in *The ASQ:SE User's Guide* for additional guidance related to these factors and for suggestions for follow-up.

   - Setting/time factors
     (e.g., Is the child's behavior the same at home as at school? Have there been any stressful events in the child's life recently?)

   - Development factors
     (e.g., Is the child's behavior related to a developmental stage or a developmental delay?)

   - Health factors
     (e.g., Is the child's behavior related to health or biological factors?)

   - Family/cultural factors
     (e.g., Is the child's behavior acceptable given cultural or family context?)

Ages & Stages Questionnaires: Social-Emotional, Squires et al.
© 2002 Paul H. Brookes Publishing Co.

7

ASQ:SE   **30 months**

Figure 12.   A completed ASQ:SE Information Summary.

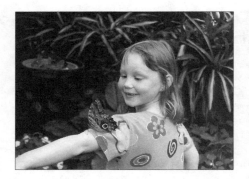

ASQ:SE Referral Criteria

The ASQ:SE questionnaires are useful only if they accurately identify children who require further evaluation (i.e., children who score above a cutoff point) and accurately exclude children who do not (i.e., children who score below a cutoff point). Questionnaire cutoff points provide an index that separates children who require referral and assessment from those who do not. A standard cutoff point, or referral criterion, for each age interval has been determined statistically using data from approximately 3,000 questionnaires. The cutoff points were derived using a variety of best-fit measures (e.g., relative or receiver operating characteristic [ROC] analyses, which are discussed further in Appendix A) and employed to obtain the ideal balance between overreferral and underreferral and to maximize sensitivity and specificity.

The recommended referral criteria outlined are based on the over- and underreferral balance. However, when assessing social-emotional delays, it is often difficult to look at assessment results as "black and white." While these criteria provide program staff with guidelines for how to interpret ASQ:SE scores, program staff must look at the larger picture prior to making decisions. Prior to making a referral, staff should consider setting/time, development, health, and family/cultural factors that may have influenced a child's score. These factors are discussed in more depth later in this chapter. In addition, the referral resources that are available to a program may require modification of a program's referral criteria. Many programs and locales may find it challenging to find services for young children with social-emotional delays. A program's access to resources may influence its referral criteria and process.

The ASQ:SE referral criteria are as follows:

- *Score is **above** the cutoff, indicating the child has a problem:* Possible referral decisions include 1) refer for diagnostic social-emotional or mental health assessment or 2) provide the parent with information and support and monitor the child using the ASQ:SE.
- *Score is **near** the cutoff, indicating the child may have a problem:* In addition to the scoring range indicated on the ASQ:SE Information Summary, programs may designate their own "questionable" range to indicate that the child's score is close to the cutoff and/or that there is a substantial parental concern (e.g., a child has a total score of 57 on the 36 month ASQ:SE, which has a cutoff score of 59, and the father has commented, "I am at the end of my rope"). Possible referral decisions may include 1) refer for diagnostic social-emotional assessment or 2) provide the parent with information and support and monitor the child using the ASQ:SE.

- *Score is **below** the cutoff, indicating the child does not have a problem:* If program resources permit, monitor the child over time using the ASQ:SE. Provide the family with information and support on any behaviors that are of concern. If you continue to have concerns about a child's social-emotional behaviors, either 1) administer an ASQ:SE with another caregiver or 2) utilize a professionally administered tool to validate or rule out concerns.

- *Parent concerns:* Follow up on any parent concerns indicated in the questionnaire. Provide information or referrals to appropriate agencies for areas of concern, for example, toilet training or age-appropriate discipline. Although a child's score may not be above or near the ASQ:SE cutoff, a decision to refer a child may be made based solely on parent concerns or the presence of a single behavior that is particularly problematic.

Professional Judgment

Given the lack of professional and financial resources currently available in the field of infant and early childhood mental health, early childhood practitioners may often feel alone and burdened with the enormous responsibility of determining the state of a young child's mental health. The ASQ:SE can assist practitioners in their decision-making process and can provide validity to referrals made to mental health professionals. However, if the results of an ASQ:SE do not validate concerns about a young child's behavior, either because the parent was unable to provide an accurate report or because the tool was not sensitive in a specific circumstance (e.g., picking up a child with subtle signs of depression), then practitioners should seek out alternative ways to identify these children and provide them with services. Options such as having an alternative caregiver complete the ASQ:SE, using a professionally administered screening tool, and administering a parent–child interaction measure are potential strategies to get information that can validate referrals. (Examples of parent–child interaction measures are included in Appendix E).

On the flip side, look carefully at ASQ:SE scores and consider the possibility of an inflated score, such as when parents mark the *sometimes* option too frequently. If your professional judgment tells you that the score may be inflated, consider the following section in this *User's Guide*, "Looking at Assessment Information in Context," which examines variables that might influence a parent's interpretation of a child's behavior. It is important to determine why an inflated score is occurring. If a referral is made and a child is determined not to have a social-emotional delay (at least to the extent that makes him or her eligible for services), it is still critically important to listen to the parent's concerns and to provide information and support related to behaviors of concern. Discuss assessment results, and gather support and information from colleagues and specialists in early childhood, family service, health, and mental health

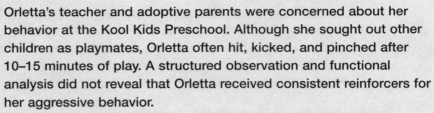

Orletta's teacher and adoptive parents were concerned about her behavior at the Kool Kids Preschool. Although she sought out other children as playmates, Orletta often hit, kicked, and pinched after 10–15 minutes of play. A structured observation and functional analysis did not reveal that Orletta received consistent reinforcers for her aggressive behavior.

The preschool director asked both Clay, Orletta's teacher, and her adoptive parents, Juan and Patrice, to complete a 48 month ASQ:SE when Orletta was 43 months old. The score on the ASQ:SE completed by Clay was 148 points, compared with a score of 85 on the questionnaire completed jointly by Orletta's parents. While the parents did not see as many aggressive behaviors at home, they were concerned about her tantrums and poor sleep habits. Because both ASQ:SE scores were above the cutoff point, Orletta's parents decided to take her to a county mental health specialist who could conduct an in-depth social-emotional assessment and make recommendations for further intervention.

fields. Infant/early childhood mental health is a new and developing field, and no practitioner should feel that he or she must have all the answers to the complex questions and situations that arise.

Looking at Assessment Information in Context

It is always important to look at assessment information in the context of other factors influencing a child's life. The ASQ:SE is designed to gather information about a child's social-emotional development and help guide referral decisions, but it is not the only information that should be considered prior to making decisions. When analyzing a young child's behavior, there are three reasons why it is critical to gather additional information other than assessment scores before making a referral decision. First, a young child's behavior may be dependent on a variety of setting/time, developmental, health, and family/cultural factors. Staff should discuss these influences to try to determine the nature of the social-emotional delays and make appropriate referrals. For example, a child with a speech delay may react emotionally when unable to communicate his or her needs (e.g., by hitting other children). Rather than immediately referring the child to a mental health professional, a more appropriate first step may be a referral to a speech-language therapist. Second, diagnostic assessments are an expensive and time-consuming process. As mentioned previously, the field of early childhood mental health is a new and growing field, but resources are lacking. The referrals that are made should be as accurate as possible and should involve appropriate and accessible services. Third, the referral process can be painful and stressful

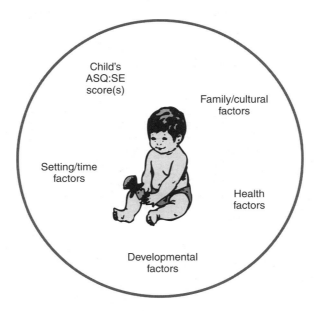

Figure 13.   Factors to consider prior to referral.

for the child and family. If preventive services can be utilized, and the child's behavior closely monitored, it may be more appropriate to continue monitoring while attempting minimal interventions or providing family support. Figure 13 provides an illustration of the factors that should be explored prior to making follow-up decisions.

A foster parent completed an ASQ:SE on Marie, a 4-year-old child in her care. Marie's total score was close to the cutoff, with the foster parent noting that Marie was wetting her pants during the day, did not seem to be happy, was not using words to get her needs met, and was not playing with other children. After the caseworker reviewed the ASQ:SE, she met and talked with the foster parent about Marie's behavior. The caseworker noted that Marie had only been in foster care for 3 weeks when the ASQ:SE was completed and felt that Marie was still adjusting to a new home. At a follow-up meeting, the foster parent indicated that Marie seemed to be more relaxed in the 2 weeks since she had completed the ASQ:SE. Together the caseworker and the foster parent decided to wait for a month before readministering the ASQ:SE and to allow Marie to settle in her new home. During that time the caseworker would enroll Marie in a therapeutic playgroup for young children who were in foster care. The caseworker advised Marie's foster parent to continue being warm and supportive and to encourage Marie to talk about her feelings.

Table 10. Factors to consider before referral, sample questions, and examples of follow-up options

Factors to consider before referral	Sample questions	Examples of follow-up options
Setting/time	Does the child act the same way at home and in child care (i.e., Is the behavior consistent across settings)? How long have the problem behaviors been occurring? Is the setting new or unfamiliar to the child/family? Where, when, and under what environmental conditions does the behavior occur? Is the child being reinforced for this behavior or gaining access to reinforcers such as a quiet corner, time alone with a teacher, or early pickup by a parent (O'Neil et al., 1997)?	Analyze environment to determine in what ways the environment is supporting or compromising the child's positive behaviors. (See Appendix E for examples of environmental assessments.) Conduct a functional behavioral analysis (LaRocque, Brown, & Johnson, 2001) to determine function of behavior(s) to child. Use results of functional analysis to create a behavior plan for child. Administer ASQ:SE to more than one parent or other caregiver to determine consistency of behavior across settings. If behavior is not consistent, consider working with parent in setting where behavior is problematic. Provide developmental information (e.g., ASQ:SE lists and activities in Appendix C), positive behavior management suggestions, and so forth. Closely monitor child's behavior; refer to a mental health professional if behavior continues to be problematic.
Development	Can the behavior be attributed to a developmental delay? Are the child's skills age level in the following domains? • Fine and gross motor • Cognitive • Personal-social • Expressive and receptive communication Is the behavior related to a developmental stage? Are individual factors (e.g., temperament) related to the child's behavior?	Screen the child using a developmental screening tool. Refer for evaluation services to Part C (early intervention) or Part B (early childhood special education) of the Individuals with Disabilities Education Act (IDEA) Amendments of 1997 (PL 105-17) if screening indicates a developmental concern. Provide developmental information (e.g., ASQ:SE lists and activities in Appendix C), positive behavior management suggestions, and so forth. Closely monitor child's behavior; refer if behavior continues to be problematic for parent.

Category	Questions	Actions
Health	Is the child's behavior related to health or biological factors? Has the child had a recent medical checkup? Have the following been considered as behavioral influences? • Hearing/vision loss • Lack of sleep or hunger • Medications or allergies • Child born addicted to drugs	Refer to primary health care providers. Address behaviors with the child's primary health care provider to determine if there is a biological/medical root to the problem. Keep in close contact with the family regarding all aspects of the child's health.
Family/cultural	Are the "problem" behaviors within the cultural norm for this child's family? What is the child's native language?	Determine if language or translation issues may be influencing parents' responses to items (e.g., misunderstanding the intent of items). Talk to family members about behaviors and whether they consider them to be problematic. Seek advice from a mental health professional who is familiar with the culture of the family to determine if behaviors are within the cultural "norm."
	Is the parent–child relationship influencing the child's ASQ:SE scores?	Use a professionally administered parent–child interaction measure (see Appendix E) to determine ways to enhance parent–child interactions. Listen carefully to parents' concerns, and provide support and help parents to understand the emotional needs of their young children. If necessary, refer to mental health specialists to assess needs and provide therapeutic services to parent–child dyad.
	Has the child been affected by stressful or traumatic events (ongoing, past, or present)? • Has the child witnessed violence in the home or in the community? • Has the child been involved in abusive or neglectful situations? • Has the child recently been moved from his or her home? • Are there family issues that are stressful (e.g., parent mental health issues, drug and alcohol issues)?	If the child is currently in a safe environment that will support prosocial behaviors, it may be appropriate to wait a short time before referring. Provide developmental information (e.g., ASQ:SE lists and activities in Appendix C), positive behavior management suggestions, and so forth. Closely monitor child's behavior; refer to a mental health professional if behavior continues to be problematic. If the child is in an unsafe environment, refer to child protective or other services. Seek advice from mental health professionals. Assist parent(s) in identifying resources and support within the community (e.g., church groups, parenting groups, drug/alcohol counseling). Refer family to mental health specialists.

Table 10 shows a list of those factors, examples of questions that could be explored if a child's score falls within a questionable range or above the cutoff on the ASQ:SE, and potential follow-up suggestions for referrals/preventive interventions. In the third column of the table are follow-up options that program staff should consider while making decisions about referrals for young children. ***These considerations are not intended to discourage professionals from making referrals for mental health evaluations or services. Rather, these considerations may help guide appropriate referrals or, when appropriate, guide preventive interventions.***

SUMMARY

Information on using, scoring, and determining follow-up criteria has been discussed in this chapter. The first phase, keeping track of the questionnaires, pertains to establishing an efficient system for mailing or presenting ASQ:SE questionnaires to families within the appropriate timeframe. The second phase, preparing the master set, includes information on individualizing and preparing the ASQ:SE for parents. The third phase, introducing the ASQ:SE, explains how to initially present the ASQ:SE system to parents. Completing the questionnaires is discussed in the fourth phase. The fifth phase, scoring the questionnaires, contains general scoring guidelines and provisions for scoring questionnaires with missing answers. The final phase, interpreting ASQ:SE results, contains guidelines for follow-up and referral based on total scores and parent comments. In addition, recommendations for additional considerations are given, taking into account the child's setting/time, development, health, and family/cultural factors.

This *User's Guide* is intended to be a reference. There are many parts that will need to be reviewed as monitoring program operations begin. Options for using questionnaires and methods for giving parents feedback may need to be tried until an appropriate set of guidelines is established for an individual program. Chapter 5 describes the final part of the ASQ:SE system, evaluating the screening and monitoring program.

5

Evaluating the Screening and Monitoring Program

ASQ:SE

This chapter focuses on evaluating the ASQ:SE screening and monitoring program. Important evaluation targets for screening and monitoring programs include 1) assessing progress in establishing and maintaining the screening and monitoring program and 2) determining the screening and monitoring program's effectiveness. Each of these evaluation targets is discussed next.

ASSESSING PROGRESS IN ESTABLISHING AND MAINTAINING THE SCREENING AND MONITORING PROGRAM

Setting up and maintaining a screening and monitoring program for a large number of children require a range of activities. The Implementation Progress Worksheet shown in Figure 14 was developed to assist program personnel in efficiently monitoring the variety of required steps necessary for initiation and maintenance of the program. The worksheet is intended to be of assistance during the initiation and early stages of developing the screening and monitoring program; however, staff may find it useful to refer back to the worksheet at designated intervals (e.g., quarterly) even after the program has been established.

The left column of the Implementation Progress Worksheet lists tasks to be completed. To the right of this column are five "action" columns: personnel needs, information needs, supplies and equipment needs, person/agency responsible, and projected date of completion. Personnel can enter in each column the indicated information for the individual steps. The final column provides four spaces to indicate the quantitative level of progress attained toward the specific step's completion. The shaded part of this column's spaces can be filled in with the month and year of each progress rating. The rating scale includes the following numerical values:

0 = *not applicable*
1 = *not begun*
2 = *partially begun or implemented*
3 = *fully completed or implemented*

ASQ:SE Implementation Progress Worksheet

Tasks	Actions						Progress rating
	Personnel needs	Information needs	Supplies and equipment needs	Person/ agency responsible	Projected date of completion		
1 Build community links/involve families							
2 Select criteria for program participation							
3 Establish program goals and objectives							
4 Determine program resources							
5 Choose management options							
6 Choose primary care and mental health providers							
7 Develop screening and monitoring activities							
8 Outline referral criteria							

Figure 14. The Implementation Progress Worksheet can be used by program personnel to monitor the tasks to be completed in the initiation and maintenance of a program using the ASQ:SE. *For progress ratings: 0 = not applicable; 1 = not begun; 2 = partially begun or implemented; 3 = fully completed or implemented.*

Tasks	Actions					Progress rating
	Personnel needs	Information needs	Supplies and equipment needs	Person/agency responsible	Projected date of completion	
9 Assemble the child file						
10 Keep track of the questionnaires						
11 Use the questionnaires						
12 Score the questionnaires						
13 Determine follow-up						

The ASQ:SE User's Guide, Squires, Bricker, and Twombly. © 2002 Paul H. Brookes Publishing Co.

(continued)

Figure 14. *(continued)*

ASQ:SE Implementation Progress Worksheet

Tasks	Actions					Progress rating
	Personnel needs	Information needs	Supplies and equipment needs	Person/ agency responsible	Projected date of completion	
14 Assess progress in establishing and maintaining the program						
15 Evaluate effectiveness						

The ASQ:SE User's Guide, Squires, Bricker, and Twombly. © 2002 Paul H. Brookes Publishing Co.

Additional program needs

1. _____

2. _____

3. _____

4. _____

5. _____

Summary: _____

_____

_____

The ASQ:SE User's Guide, Squires, Bricker, and Twombly. © 2002 Paul H. Brookes Publishing Co.

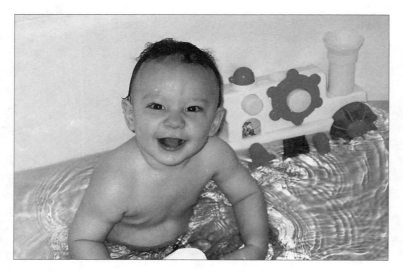

During initial start-up, program staff may want to evaluate their progress weekly using the Implementation Progress Worksheet. Later, monthly or quarterly evaluations of progress may be sufficient. Tasks to evaluate will change as the program matures and as more children are being monitored. As program objectives are modified, it may be necessary to begin a new worksheet reflecting these new objectives.

For example, in the case study in Chapter 3 that described how Four Corners Head Start developed a two-level system of ASQ:SE distribution, the procedures for follow-up may need to be modified. The mental health specialist may be unable to contact all 106 parents who did not return the questionnaire. The procedure may need to be modified so that the classroom teacher contacts a portion of parents and the mental health coordinator concentrates on those deemed at highest risk.

Although most programs will strive for ratings of 3 on most tasks, there may be instances in which a rating of 2 is sufficient. Limited resources, lower priority, or modification of tasks may be reasons for these lower ratings. If a modification occurs, tasks should be rewritten and reevaluated.

To begin, staff first establish their personnel resources, which includes having the program director and two coordinators conduct a cost analysis of resources needed for mail-out methods only versus home visits for completion of the first ASQ:SE followed by the mail-out method for subsequent questionnaires. The cost analysis of home visiting (e.g., personnel, supplies, mileage) and of the mail-out method (e.g., postage stamps, supplies, clerical time, computer and software for word processing, letterhead stationery, telephone with two lines) will assist in the completion of Task 5, choosing management options. The director's time to complete the study is approximately 10 hours; the two coordinators' time approximately 8 hours each, for 16 hours total of coordinator time.

Staff also need to decide the person/agency responsible for implementing the screening and monitoring system. Coordinators will have the responsibility of gathering information from personnel timesheets for home visitors and clerical staff as well as summarizing materials and supplies costs.

DETERMINE THE SCREENING AND
MONITORING PROGRAM'S EFFECTIVENESS

Every screening and monitoring program, even one with limited resources, should conduct some form of evaluation to determine the effectiveness of the program and the procedures being used. How extensively each of these areas can be evaluated will depend on the program's resources and staff expertise. The following areas of evaluation are recommended:

- ASQ:SE return rate
- Parent feedback
- Effectiveness of ASQ:SE in accurately identifying children
- Feedback from personnel
- Feedback from collaborating agencies

ASQ:SE Return Rate

If the program mails the ASQ:SE to families, a record of the return rate should be maintained and calculated on a regular basis (e.g., every 6 months). If a program has less than a 60% return rate, modification of procedures should be considered.

Parent Feedback

Feedback from parents should be sought at least yearly. A simple, short survey can be devised and included with a questionnaire once a year (e.g., at 12, 24, 36, 48, and 60 months). Figure 15 is an example of such a survey.

Effectiveness of ASQ:SE in Accurately Identifying Children

To examine the effectiveness of the questionnaires, it is imperative to keep records of the number of children identified as needing further assessment and the outcome of their subsequent assessments. By recording this information, it is possible to determine the percentage of children accurately identified by the questionnaires as having social-emotional problems and those who were incorrectly recommended for further evaluation. These calculations provide information on the sensitivity and over-referral rates for the group of children being monitored.[1] Providing information on the effectiveness of a screening program may help personnel in a variety of ways. First, data on the effectiveness of the screening program may be requested and appreciated by funding sources. Second, additional information may be provided about the monitoring of implementation goals. For example, a program may project a screening rate of 10% prior

---

[1]Specificity and underreferral rates cannot be calculated unless a program conducts follow-up assessments with children who are not identified by the questionnaires as needing further assessment, as well as with children identified as needing further assessment.

ASQ:SE

Dear Parent,

Would you please take a few minutes to evaluate the ASQ:SE? We appreciate your participation in our program and hope that our services have been helpful to you.

1. Were the questionnaires appropriate for your child?
    yes ☐   no ☐
    Comments:

2. Were the questionnaires useful to complete?
    yes ☐   no ☐
    Comments:

3. Were any items unclear or difficult to understand?
    yes ☐   no ☐
    If yes, which items?

    Comments:

4. Would you like more information on social-emotional development?
    yes ☐   no ☐
    If yes, which areas?

    Comments:

5. Would you like to fill out another questionnaire as your child gets older?
    yes ☐   no ☐
    Comments:

We welcome any further comments you have about the questionnaires. Feel free to write on the back of this form.

The ASQ:SE User's Guide, Squires, Bricker, and Twombly. © 2002 Paul H. Brookes Publishing Co.

Figure 15.   An example of a feedback form sent to parents participating in a monitoring program. Such a survey should be distributed at least once a year, if possible. A Spanish translation of this form is provided in Appendix G.

to initiation of the screening and monitoring program. Following the first year, program staff can calculate the actual screening rate and compare it with the 10% projection. If the program's goal of 10% is not realized (i.e., percentage screened is significantly higher or lower than the anticipated screening rate), the criteria used to include children in the program may need to be modified. Figure 16 provides a contingency table and formulas for calculating the percentage of children appropriately identified as needing further assessment, as well as the sensitivity, specificity, overreferral and underreferral rates, and positive predictive value.

Feedback from Personnel

It is important to seek formal or informal feedback from personnel using the questionnaires, learning from them which program procedures work

		Follow-up assessment	
		Intervention needs	No intervention needs
Ages & Stages Questionnaires: Social-Emotional	At risk; identified as needing further assessment	True positives A	False positives (overreferral) B
	Okay; not identified	False negatives (underreferral) C	True negatives D

Percent of children identified as needing further assessment:

$$\frac{A + B}{A + B + C + D}$$

Sensitivity The proportion of children correctly identified by the questionnaires as needing further assessment:

$$\frac{A}{A + C}$$

Specificity The proportion of children correctly identified by the questionnaires as developing typically:

$$\frac{D}{B + D}$$

Overreferral The proportion of children (of the total number of children for whom a questionnaire was completed) incorrectly identified by the questionnaires as needing further assessment:

$$\frac{B}{A + B + C + D}$$

Underreferral The proportion of children (of the total number of children for whom a questionnaire was completed) incorrectly excluded by the questionnaires:

$$\frac{C}{A + B + C + D}$$

Positive predictive value The proportion of children identified by the questionnaires as needing further assessment who will, in fact, have intervention needs:

$$\frac{A}{A + B}$$

Figure 16.   Contingency table, definitions, and formulas for evaluating the effectiveness of the ASQ:SE monitoring program.

well and which ones do not. The ASQ:SE system is flexible, and program personnel can and should make adjustments in its use to ensure efficient and effective application. At least once a year, staff should meet to examine ways to improve the activities associated with their screening and monitoring program.

A completed Implementation Progress Worksheet is presented in Figure 17 for the Steps-Ahead program. After 6 months, the Steps-Ahead staff reviewed their progress in completing implementation tasks (e.g., they checked whether the goals and objectives, program resources, and method-of-use tasks were implemented and had met projected dates of completion). For the first task, building community links/involving parents, staff felt positive about their relationships with families. However, they wanted to add parents to the management team and needed more time to assess how this could best be implemented. The selecting criteria for participation, involving parents, and determining referral criteria tasks were only partially implemented, receiving ratings of 2. Criteria for participation had been determined; however, there had not been an adequate number of children to evaluate outcomes. Therefore, staff decided to use the selection criteria on an experimental basis for 3 more months, keeping careful records on numbers of children being screened.

The sixth task, involving primary health and mental health care providers, had not yet been implemented. It was felt that additional members were needed on the advisory board to assist in making physician contacts, especially for rural areas. When additional board members agree to serve, this task can be implemented.

Regarding the tasks for using and scoring the questionnaires, all clerical and office tasks related to setting up and maintaining child files had been completed. The computer database system for Steps-Ahead had been modified so that the ASQ:SE was included in the tickler system along with the ASQ.

Home visitors had used the ASQ:SE on 20 children and believed they needed additional time to determine if follow-up procedures were effective. Therefore, the task of determining follow-up received a rating of 2. The Steps-Ahead staff wanted to use the questionnaires with at least 50 families and to have referred at least 6 children before they evaluated the effectiveness of follow-up procedures.

ASQ:SE Implementation Progress Worksheet

| Tasks | Actions | | | | | | Progress rating | |
	Personnel needs	Information needs	Supplies and equipment needs	Person/ agency responsible	Projected date of completion	9/1	12/1	
1 Build community links/involve families	Advisory board, parent representatives, coordinators, Local Early Intervention Interagency Coordinating Council (LICC)	Community resources	Computer database software, web access for agency directories	Directors, coordinators	6/1	2		
2 Select criteria for program participation	Physicians, counselors on advisory board; 2 meetings	Risk criteria from research studies, LICC recommendations	Library, computer search capabilities	Director to assist with search and scheduling meetings	7/1	2		
3 Establish program goals and objectives	Schedule four 2-hour staff meetings to discuss, outline	State and federal regulations, community resources	Large writing paper and pens	Director	6/1	3		
4 Determine program resources	Social workers, advisory board; director, coordinators	Available resources and in-kind contributions	Computer software for word processor, database	Director	7/1	3		
5 Choose management options	Coordinators	Available resources (#4), needs and characteristics of parents	Copy machine, computer tickler system	Director	8/1	3		
6 Choose primary care and mental health providers	Physicians, counselors, therapists on advisory board	Names of physicians at HMOs, social workers and counselors	Mailing labels, telephone, word processor	Advisory board— physician contacts, clerical staff— letters	2/1	1		
7 Develop screening and monitoring activities	Staff; weekly meetings	Available resources (#4), referral resources (#1), management plan (#5)	Computer, software, secretarial support	Director	8/1	2		
8 Outline referral criteria	Advisory board, coordinators, social workers	List of community resources for evaluation, cutoffs from User's Guide	Word processor	Director	2/1	2		

The ASQ:SE User's Guide, Squires, Bricker, and Twombly. © 2002 Paul H. Brookes Publishing Co.

(continued)

Figure 17.   Implementation Progress Worksheet completed by Steps-Ahead staff 6 months after the initiation of a screening and monitoring program using the ASQ:SE.

Figure 17. *(continued)*

ASQ:SE Implementation Progress Worksheet

Tasks	Actions					Projected date of completion	Progress rating	
	Personnel needs	Information needs	Supplies and equipment needs	Person/ agency responsible			9/1	12/1
9 Assemble the child file	Clerical staff	ID # system, family information	File folders, labels	Clerical staff		8/1	3	
10 Keep track of the questionnaires	Social workers, home visitors	Child's date of birth and family information	Computer tickler system	Social workers, home visitors		8/1	3	
11 Use the questionnaires	Social workers, home visitors	Directions from The ASQ:SE User's Guide	ASQ:SE at each interval, letters from User's Guide	Social workers, home visitors		8/1	3	
12 Score the questionnaires	Social workers, home visitors	Scoring directions from The ASQ:SE User's Guide	Information Summary Sheets from ASQ:SE	Social workers, home visitors		8/1	3	
13 Determine follow-up	Social workers, home visitors, counselors	Referral criteria (#8), availability of community evaluation and support services	List of community resources, telephone numbers	Social workers— contacts with referral sources, Director— contacts with physicians		9/1	2	

The ASQ:SE User's Guide, Squires, Bricker, and Twombly. © 2002 Paul H. Brookes Publishing Co.

| Tasks | Actions | | | | | Progress rating | |
	Personnel needs	Information needs	Supplies and equipment needs	Person/agency responsible	Projected date of completion	9/1	12/1
14 Assess progress in establishing and maintaining the program	Monthly staff meetings	Progress worksheet	Clerical supplies, computer	Director	9/1—Evaluate overall progress	2	
15 Evaluate effectiveness	Social workers, counselors, home visitors, Director	Outcomes from child evaluations, public school placements for 4- to 5-year-olds	Computer, calculator, formulas from The ASQ:SE User's Guide	Director	9/1	2	

(continued)

The ASQ:SE User's Guide, Squires, Bricker, and Twombly. © 2002 Paul H. Brookes Publishing Co.

Figure 17. *(continued)*

ASQ:SE Implementation Progress Worksheet

Additional program needs

1. *Ensure links between Steps-Ahead and early intervention programs so that Steps-Ahead can find out what the outcomes are for children referred for social-emotional and/or mental health assessment.*

2. *Identify and ask two parents and one child psychiatrist or psychologist to join the advisory board, as well as one rural physician.*

3. *Develop and circulate parent satisfaction questionnaire.*

4. _____

5. _____

Summary: _____

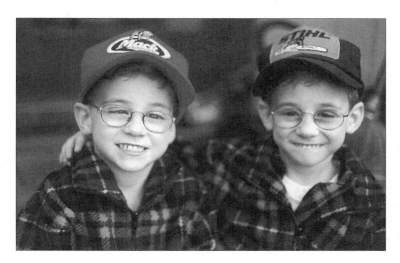

Feedback from Collaborating Agencies

If more than one agency is involved in the screening and monitoring program, it may be important to determine the effectiveness of the collaboration between agencies. Formal mechanisms should be established (e.g., annual meetings) to ensure that communication between agencies is sufficient and effective. Ensuring that methods for resolving conflicts are in place and working is also important.

SUMMARY

Evaluating the screening and monitoring program involves two targets—assessing progress in establishing and maintaining the screening and monitoring program and determining the screening and monitoring program's effectiveness. Progress can be assessed by monitoring project staff accomplishments during monthly or quarterly staff meetings and should not require extensive information or data that go beyond day-to-day operations of the program. Determination of the system's effectiveness is also of prime importance. Information may be needed from outside referral agencies to determine child evaluation outcomes. These data are necessary in order to determine whether the program is effective: Are the right children being identified for further evaluation? Are they then referred for early intervention services? Evaluation of the monitoring program should be ongoing, and revision of steps and activities will be necessary as the program grows and changes.

References

Abidin, R.R. (n.d.). *Parenting Stress Index–3* (3rd ed.). Circle Pines, MN: American Guidance Service.

Achenbach, T. (1991). *Manual for the Child Behavior Checklist/4–18 and 1991 profile.* Burlington: University of Vermont, Department of Psychiatry.

Achenbach, T., & Rescorla, L. (2000). *Manual for the ASEBA preschool forms and profiles.* Burlington, VT: ASEBA.

Bagnato, S.J., Neisworth, J.T., Salvia, J., & Hunt, F.M. (1999). *Temperamental and Atypical Behavior Scale (TABS): Early Childhood Indicators of Developmental Dysfunction.* Baltimore: Paul H. Brookes Publishing Co.

Bandura, A. (1997). *Self-efficacy: The exercise of control.* New York: W.H. Freeman.

Bost, K., Vaughn, B., Washington, W., Cielinski, K., & Bradbard, M. (1998). Social competence, social support, and attachment: Demarcation of construct domains, measurement, and paths of influence for preschool children attending Head Start. *Child Development, 69*(1), 192–218.

Bricker, D., & Squires, J. (with Mounts, L., Potter, L., Nickel, R., Twombly, E., & Farrell, J.). (1999). *Ages & Stages Questionnaires (ASQ): A Parent-Completed, Child-Monitoring System* (2nd ed.). Baltimore: Paul H. Brookes Publishing Co.

Bricker, D., Squires, J., & Mounts, L. (with Potter, L., Nickel, R., & Farrell, J.). (1995). *Ages & Stages Questionnaires (ASQ): A Parent-Completed, Child-Monitoring System.* Baltimore: Paul H. Brookes Publishing Co.

Briggs-Gowan, M.J., & Carter, A.S. (1998). Preliminary acceptability and psychometrics of the Infant-Toddler Social and Emotional Assessment (ITSEA): A new adult-report questionnaire. *Infant Mental Health Journal, 19*(4), 422–445.

Bureau of the Census. (2001, April). *PHC-T-1: Population by race and Hispanic or Latino origin* [On-line], Available: http://www.census.gov.

Campos, J., Mumme, D., Kermoina, R., & Campos, R. (1994). A functionalist perspective on the nature of emotion. *Monographs of the Society for Research in Child Development, 59*(2–3, Serial No. 240), 284–303.

Carey, W., & McDevitt, S. (n.d.). *Carey Temperament Scales (CTS).* Scottsdale, AZ: Behavioral-Developmental Initiatives.

Chan, B., & Taylor, N. (1998).The follow along program cost analysis in southwest Minnesota. *Infants and Young Children, 10*(4), 71–79.

Cicchetti, D. (1993). Developmental psychology: Reactions, reflections, projections. *Developmental Review, 13,* 471–502

Cicchetti, D., & Toth, S.L. (2000). Child maltreatment in the early years of life. In J.D. Osofsky & H.E. Fitzgerald (Eds.), *WAIMH handbook of infant mental health: Vol. 4. Infant mental health in groups at high risk* (pp. 255–294). New York: John Wiley & Sons.

Conners, C.K. (1997). *Conners' Rating Scale* (Rev. ed.). North Tonawanda, NY: Multi-Health Systems.

DeGangi, G., & Greenspan, S. (2000). Functional emotional assessment scale. In G. DeGangi, *Pediatric disorders of regulation in affect and behavior: A therapist's guide to assessment and treatment* (pp. 341–360). San Diego: Academic Press.

DeGangi, G., Poisson, S., Sickel, R., & Wiener, A.S. (1999). *Infant/Toddler Symptom Checklist.* Austin, TX: Therapy Skill Builders.

Devereux Foundation. (1998). *Devereux Early Childhood Assessment Program (DECA).* Lewisville, NC: Kaplan Companies.

Dishion, T., French, D., & Patterson, G. (1995). The development and ecology of antisocial behavior. In D. Cicchetti & D. Cohen (Eds.), *Developmental psychopathology: Vol. 2. Risk, disorder, and adaptation* (pp. 388–394). New York: John Wiley & Sons.

Duncan, G., & Brooks-Gunn, J. (2000). Family, poverty, welfare reform, and child development. *Child Development, 71*(1), 188–196.

Emde, R.N., Korfmacher, J., & Kubicek, L.F. (2000). Toward a theory of early relationship-based intervention. In J.D. Osofsky & H.E. Fitzgerald (Eds.), *WAIMH handbook of infant mental health: Vol. 2. Early intervention, evaluation, and assessment* (pp. 3–24). New York: John Wiley & Sons.

Eyberg, S. (n.d.). *Eyberg Child Behavior Inventory.* Odessa, FL: Psychological Assessment Resources, Inc.

Feil, E., Walker, H., & Severson, H. (1995). The early screening project for young children with behavior problems. *Journal of Emotional and Behavioral Disorders, 3*(4), 194–202.

Finello, K.M., & Poulsen, M.K. (1996). *Behavioral Assessment of Baby's Emotional and Social Style (BABES).* Los Angeles: California School of Professional Psychology–Los Angeles.

Fox, N.A. (Ed.). (1994). The development of emotion regulation: Biological and behavioral considerations. *Monographs of the Society for Research in Child Development, 59*(2–3, Serial No. 240), 103–107.

Garbarino, J., & Ganzel, B. (2000). The human ecology of early risk. In J.P. Shonkoff & S.J. Meisels (Eds.), *Handbook of early childhood intervention* (2nd ed., pp. 76–93). New York: Cambridge University Press.

Greenspan, S., & Wieder, S. (1993). Regulation disorders. In C.H. Zeanah (Ed.), *Handbook of infant mental health* (pp. 280–290). New York: Guilford Press.

Gresham, F.M., & Elliott, S.N. (n.d.). *Social Skills Rating System (SSRS).* Circle Pines, MN: American Guidance Service.

Guralnick, M.J. (Ed.). (1997). *The effectiveness of early intervention.* Baltimore: Paul H. Brookes Publishing Co.

Hart, B., & Risley, T.R. (1995). *Meaningful differences in the everyday lives of young American children.* Baltimore: Paul H. Brookes Publishing Co.

Hart, B., & Risley, T.R. (1999). *The social world of children learning to talk.* Baltimore: Paul H. Brookes Publishing Co.

Individuals with Disabilities Education Act (IDEA) Amendments of 1997, PL 105-17, 20 U.S.C. §§ 1400 *et seq.*

Kazdin, A. (1987). Treatment of antisocial behavior in children: Current status and future directions. *Psychological Bulletin,102*(2), 187–203.

Knitzer, J. (2000). Early childhood mental health services: A policy and systems development perspective. In J.P. Shonkoff & S.J. Meisels (Eds.), *Handbook of early childhood intervention* (2nd ed., pp. 416–438). New York: Cambridge University Press.

LaRocque, M., Brown, S.E., & Johnson, K.L. (2001). Functional behavioral assessments and intervention plans in early intervention settings. *Infants and Young Children, 13*(3), 59–68.

Lyons-Ruth, K., Alpern L., & Repacholi, B. (1993). Disorganized infant attachment classification and maternal psychosocial problems as predictors of hostile-aggressive behavior in the preschool classroom. *Child Development, 64,* 572–585.

Merrell, K. (1994). *Manual for the Preschool and Kindergarten Behavior Scale (PKBS).* Austin, TX: PRO-ED.

O'Neil, R.E., Horner, R.H., Albin, R.W., Sprague, J.R., Storkey, K., & Newton, J.S. (1997). *Functional assessment and program development for problem behavior: A practical handbook* (2nd ed.). Pacific Grove, CA: Brooks/Cole Thomson Learning.

Osofsky, J.D., & Fitzgerald, H.E. (Eds.). (2000). *WAIMH handbook of infant mental health: Vol. 4. Infant mental health in groups at high risk.* New York: John Wiley & Sons.

Osofsky, J.D., & Thompson, M.D. (2000). Adaptive and maladaptive parenting: Perspectives on risk and protective factors. In J.P. Shonkoff & S.J. Meisels (Eds.), *Handbook of early childhood intervention* (2nd ed., pp. 54–75). New York: Cambridge University Press.

Patterson, G.R., Reid, B., & Dishion, T.J. (1992). *Antisocial boys.* Eugene, OR: Castalia.

Provence, S., & Apfel, N.A. (2001). *Infant-Toddler and Family Instrument (ITFI).* Baltimore: Paul H. Brookes Publishing Co.

Raver, C.C., & Zigler, E.F. (1997). Social competence: An untapped dimension in evaluating Head Start's success. *Early Childhood Quarterly, 12,* 363–385.

Reid, J. (1993). Prevention of conduct disorder before and after school entry: Relating intervention to developmental findings. *Developmental and Social Psychology, 5,* 241–260.

Reynolds, C., & Kamphaus, R. (1992). *Behavioral Assessment System for Children (BASC).* Circle Pines, MN: American Guidance Service.

Rogosch, F.A., Cicchetti, D., Shields, A., & Toth, S. (1996). Parental dysfunction in child maltreatment. In M. Bornstein (Ed.), *Handbook of parenting* (Vol. 4, pp. 127–162). Mahwah, NJ: Lawrence Erlbaum Associates.

Sameroff, A. (2000). Ecological perspectives on developmental risk. In J.D. Osofsky & H.E. Fitzgerald (Eds.), *WAIMH handbook of infant mental health: Vol. 4. Infant mental health in groups at high risk* (pp. 1–33). New York: John Wiley & Sons.

Sameroff, A.J., & Fiese, B.H. (2000). Transactional regulation: The developmental ecology of early intervention. In J.P. Shonkoff & S.J. Meisels (Eds.), *Handbook of early childhood intervention* (2nd ed., pp. 135–159). New York: Cambridge University Press.

Sameroff, A.J., Seifer, R., Baldwin, A., & Baldwin, C. (1994). Stability of intelligence from preschool to adolescence: The influence of social and family risk factors. *Child Development, 64,* 80–97.

Sparrow, S., Balla, D., & Cicchetti, D. (1998). *Vineland Social-Emotional Early Childhood Scale (SEEC).* Circle Pines, MN: American Guidance Service.

Sprague, S., & Walker, H. (2000). Early identification and intervention for youth with antisocial and violent behavior. *Exceptional Children, 66*(3), 367–379.

Squires, J., Potter, L., & Bricker, D. (1999). *The ASQ user's guide for the Ages & Stages Questionnaires: A Parent-Completed, Child-Monitoring System* (2nd ed.). Baltimore: Paul H. Brookes Publishing Co.

Thompson, R.A. (1994). Emotion regulation: A theme in search of definition. *Monographs of the Society for Research in Child Development, 59*(2–3, Serial No. 240), 250–283.

Walker, H.M., Irvin, L.K., & Sprague, J.R. (1997, Fall). Violence prevention and school safety issues, problems, approaches, and recommended solutions. *Oregon School Study Council Bulletin, 41*(1).

Walker, H.M., Kavanagh, K., Stiller, B., Golly, A., Severson, H., & Feil, E. (1998). Early intervention for antisocial behavior. *Journal of Emotional and Behavioral Disorders, 6*(2), 66–80.

Walker, H.M., Severson, H.H., & Feil, E. (1995). *Early Screening Project.* Longmont, CO: Sopris West.

Waters, E., & Sroufe, L.A. (1983). Social competence as a developmental construct. *Developmental Review, 3,* 79–97.

Weinberg, K., & Tronick, E.Z. (1997). Maternal depression and infant maladjustment: A failure of mutual regulation. In J. Noshpitz, S. Greenspan, J.D. Osofsky, & S. Weider (Eds.), *Handbook of child and adolescent psychiatry* (Vol. 1, pp. 177–190). New York: John Wiley & Sons.

Wittmer, D., Doll, B., & Strain, P. (1996). Social and emotional development in early childhood: The identification of competence and disabilities. *Journal of Early Intervention, 20*(4), 299–318.

Zeanah, C.H. (Ed.). (2000). *Handbook of infant mental health* (2nd ed.). New York: Guilford Press.

Zeitlin, S., Williamson, G.G., & Szczepanski, M. (1988). *Early Coping Inventory (ECI).* Bensenville, IL: Scholastic Testing Service.

ZERO TO THREE. (1994). *Diagnostic classification: 0–3. Diagnostic classification of mental health and developmental disorders of infancy and early childhood.* Arlington, VA: Author.

Appendixes

ASQ:SE

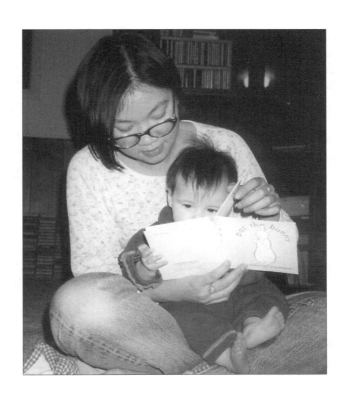

Technical Report on ASQ:SE

ASQ:SE

Information relating to the development and psychometric studies completed on the ASQ:SE is contained in this appendix. In the first section, development of the ASQ:SE system, including item selection, is addressed, followed by a description of the initial field-test version. The second section describes the participants; the measures used to collect demographic, reliability, and validity data from the normative sample; and the procedures used to collect demographic and psychometric data. Third, demographic characteristics of the ASQ:SE research sample are described. Fourth, psychometric findings are reported, including internal consistency, test–retest reliability, concurrent validity, and known groups (criterion-referenced) validity. Findings on the utility of the ASQ:SE are reported in the fifth section.

DEVELOPMENT OF THE ASQ:SE

Item Selection

ASQ:SE items were developed using a variety of sources, including standardized social-emotional and developmental assessments, textbooks and other resources in developmental and abnormal psychology, education and intervention resources, and language and communication materials. Items were created using the following criteria:

1. Items need to be representative of critical adaptive and maladaptive behaviors at the targeted age intervals.
2. Items are easy for parents to understand and recognize.
3. Items are appropriate for a variety of cultural groups and families.

Each item was written using common words that did not exceed a sixth-grade reading level. When possible, quantitative descriptors (e.g., 15 minutes, within a 24-hour period) and concrete examples (e.g., kicks, bites other children) were provided to assist with interpretation of the item meanings.

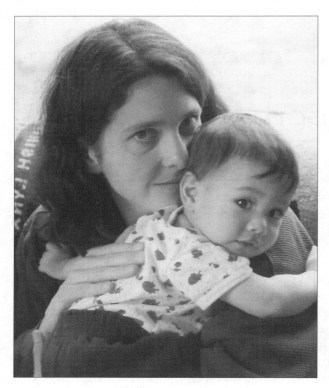

Field-Test Version

Once items were written, they were assembled into a field-test version, which was titled the *Behavior-Ages & Stages Questionnaires* (B-ASQ; Squires, Bricker, Twombly, Yockelson, & Kim, 1996). The field-test version contained seven age intervals. The number of items per interval varied from 21 items at 6 months to 33 items at 48 months. The items in this field-test version were reviewed by experts in psychology, psychiatry, education, early childhood development, pediatrics, nursing, and mental health. Experts provided feedback on the appropriateness of items, ease of understanding items, scoring format, and content validity.

Concurrently, practitioners in approximately 50 programs across the United States used the B-ASQ with a diverse population of young children and parents, including the following:

- Families served by Healthy Start in Hawaii and Oregon
- Inner-city families in Cincinnati, Ohio; Portland, Oregon; and San Francisco, California
- Families served by Head Start or Migrant Head Start in California, Texas, and Washington State
- Families with young children identified with social and emotional problems in Arizona, California, Oregon, Utah, and Washington State

Utility questionnaires completed by service providers and parents provided feedback on the clarity of item meaning, appropriateness of items, missing content, and suggestions for revisions or additions of items.

Final Version

Based on the input gathered from experts, parents, and practitioners, and on preliminary data analyses, the B-ASQ was revised and renamed the *Ages & Stages Questionnaires: Social-Emotional (ASQ:SE)*. Five types of changes were made to the field-test version. First, items with overlapping and similar content were combined. Second, items were added to fill content gaps (e.g., items were added to target so-called "red flags" for autism [Filipek, Accardo, Ashwall, et al. 2000; Filipek, Accardo, Baranek, et al.,

1999]). Third, some items were reworded to be more understandable for parents. Fourth, format changes were made to improve readability and utility for parents. Finally, a questionnaire was added at 60 months so that the questionnaire system could cover the entire infant through pre-school age span.

The final English version of the ASQ:SE was translated into Spanish by Spanish-speaking personnel from a Migrant Head Start program in Oregon. The Spanish translation was used with 153 children whose families were non-English speakers. These translated questionnaires were not included in ASQ:SE reliability or validity analyses.

DATA COLLECTION PROCEDURES

Participant Recruitment

Children between the ages of 3 and 66 months and their parents were recruited for a national normative study of the ASQ:SE. Several recruiting methods were used, including gathering information from birth announcements and advertisements in Pacific Northwest newspapers; sending recruitment letters to child care providers in California and Oregon; making personal contacts with personnel in agencies serving high-risk families and young children with disabilities in California, Connecticut, Florida, Hawaii, Michigan, North Carolina, Ohio, and Oregon; and setting up information booths at children's fairs and shopping malls in Oregon and Washington State. An attempt was made to stratify the normative sample so that children and families would be representative of the U.S. population in terms of ethnicity, geographic region, parent education, income, and sex of children (Bureau of the Census, 2000a, 2000b, 2001). Recruitment letters and research protocols were approved by the University of Oregon Human Subjects Compliance Committee prior to the beginning of the study.

Measures

Three types of measures were used to collect data on the normative sample: a demographic form, the ASQ:SE questionnaires for each age interval, and two social-emotional measures with established psychometric properties (i.e., Child Behavior Checklist [CBCL; Achenbach, 1991, 1992] and Vineland Social-Emotional Early Childhood Scale [SEEC; Sparrow, Balla, & Cicchetti, 1998]). The demographic form asked parents to provide information on the child's age, gender, and ethnicity, as well as information on the mother's education level and family income.

The ASQ:SE covers eight age intervals from 6 to 60 months and is described previously in Chapter 1 of this *User's Guide*. The questionnaires are designed to be completed by parents or caregivers who can provide information on a child's social-emotional competence.

To assess the concurrent validity of the ASQ:SE, a sample of children was given the CBCL or the SEEC. Additional children with a formal diagnosis of "social-emotional disability" were also recruited. These procedures are described next.

Procedures

Parents who indicated a willingness to participate in the study were given a packet of materials containing a consent form, ASQ:SE questionnaire, and demographic form. Packets were distributed in four ways: by mail (e.g., parents contacted through birth announcements and newspaper advertisements), by preschool teachers directly to parents, by personnel in agencies serving young children and families who distributed them to interested parents, and by research personnel directly to parents (e.g., at shopping malls and children's fairs). When parents received a packet, they were asked to return the completed forms within 1 week. If parents did not return the packets, telephone calls were made or reminder notes were sent.

After the packets were returned, a random sample of parents were contacted by telephone and asked if they would be willing to complete a second set of questionnaires and/or have their child participate in a direct assessment. Parents who agreed were given two options according to the age of their child: 1) complete a second ASQ:SE and/or the CBCL at home, to be returned in a pre-stamped envelope within 1 week (for children 24–66 months of age), or 2) permit an assessment of their child with one of two trained examiners using the SEEC in the family's home or another convenient location (for children 3–24 months of age). Prior to these assessments, the two trained examiners had established interrater reliability exceeding 95%.

Data from parental completion of the second ASQ:SE were used to examine test–retest reliability, while data gathered from parents completing the CBCL and from trained examiners' completion of the SEEC were used to examine the validity of the ASQ:SE. As the packets were returned, information from the demographic form and questionnaires as well as the CBCL and SEEC results were entered into computer files for analyses.

DEMOGRAPHIC CHARACTERISTICS OF NORMATIVE SAMPLE

Children between the ages of 3 and 66 months were recruited to examine the psychometric properties of the ASQ:SE. Approximately 10% were recruited through birth announcements in newspapers; 10% through newspaper advertisements; 30% through agency personnel who attended national conferences and agreed to field test the ASQ:SE; 35% through early intervention/early childhood special education centers and parent education programs; and 15% through children's fairs or booths at shopping malls. Data for demographic variables such as ethnicity, family income, and mother's education level were not always provided by parents for a variety of reasons (e.g., privacy). The number of children with missing data and the type of missing data are noted for each analysis.

Table A1.   Number of questionnaires and gender distribution by ASQ:SE age interval

ASQ:SE age interval	Number of questionnaires		
	Total	Males	Females
6 month	355	176	175
12 month	375	189	180
18 month	323	146	172
24 month	471	249	219
30 month	298	169	126
36 month	425	199	207
48 month	457	215	221
60 month	310	153	154
Overall	3,014[a]	1,496[a]	1,454[a]

[a]Gender data missing for 64 children.

The total number of ASQ:SE assessments completed on children was 3,014. The distribution of these questionnaires by age interval and gender is shown in Table A1. The ASQ:SE total sample included 2,633 children (87%) whose families contributed at least one completed questionnaire and 381 (13%) whose families contributed two or more questionnaires at different age intervals (e.g., questionnaires at 6 and 12 months). Of the 381 families that completed two or more questionnaires, 59 contributed four or more questionnaires.

Table A2 contains a comparison of Bureau of the Census (2001) counts of the ethnic distribution with those of the ASQ:SE normative sample. There appears to be an apparent underrepresentation of Caucasians and an overrepresentation of individuals with mixed ethnicity. This is not a straightforward comparison, given the large numbers of individuals who identified themselves as mixed ethnicity.

According to data provided by the Bureau of the Census (2001), the ASQ:SE normative sample has a higher percentage of well-educated mothers than found generally in the United States, as shown in Table A3, although again these comparisons are not straightforward given differing categories of analysis. A comparison between the U.S. Census data and the ASQ:SE sample on income level indicates the ASQ:SE sample was

Table A2.   Ethnicity comparison of ASQ:SE normative sample (N = 2,952) with 2000 Census estimates

Ethnic category	Percentage		Percentage point difference
	ASQ:SE normative sample	2000 U.S. Census[a]	
Caucasian	58.9	69.1	−10.2
African American	8.9	12.1	−3.2
Hispanic	8.6	12.5	−3.9
Asian/Pacific Islander	6.3	3.7	+2.6
Native American	1.1	0.7	+0.4
Mixed ethnicity	16.0	1.6	+14.4

Note: Ethnicity data missing for 62 children.
[a]Bureau of the Census (2001).

Table A3. Mother's education level comparison of ASQ:SE normative sample (*N* = 2,863) with 2000 Census figures

	Percentage		
Level of education	ASQ:SE normative sample	2000 U.S. Census[a]	Percentage point difference
Less than high school graduation	13.0	20.9	−7.9
High school graduation or equivalent	47.4	51.0	−3.6
Associate degree	11.9	7.5	+4.4
4-year college degree or above	25.3	20.6	+4.7
Don't know	2.4	—[b]	—

Note: Mother's level of education data missing for 151 children.

[a]Bureau of the Census (2000b).

[b]U.S. Census does not include a "Don't know" category.

composed of a higher percentage of families with lower incomes than is found in the general population, as shown in Table A4.

Data taken from the demographic form permitted dividing the ASQ:SE normative sample into four groups according to the children's developmental status: 1) no risk (i.e., children with one or no identified environmental/medical risk factors), 2) at risk (i.e., children with two or more risk factors), 3) developmental disability (i.e., children with established developmental disabilities who were receiving early intervention/ early childhood special education services through IDEA), and 4) social-emotional disability (i.e., children with identified social-emotional disabilities, according to IDEA Part B eligibility guidelines and the *Diagnostic and Statistical Manual of Mental Disorders, Fourth Edition* [DSM-IV; American Psychiatric Association, 1994], diagnostic classifications). Variables used to determine level of risk for the first two groups included the following:

1. Family income less than $12,000
2. Mother less than 18 years old when child was born
3. Mother's level of education less than high school graduation
4. Involvement of child protective services with family
5. Child in foster care
6. Birth weight less than 3 pounds, 5 ounces

Table A5 presents the number of children by developmental status in the normative sample.

PSYCHOMETRIC FINDINGS

The following sections discuss how the cutoff scores for the ASQ:SE were developed. In addition, data collected from subgroups of the normative sample used to examine the internal consistency, test–retest, concurrent validity, known groups validity, and utility of the ASQ:SE are presented.

Table A4.   Family income level comparison of ASQ:SE normative sample (N = 1,992) with 1999 Bureau of the Census estimates

	ASQ:SE	1999 Bureau of the Census estimates		
Income category	Percentage of normative sample	Income category[a]	Percentage of population	Percentage point difference
$0–12,000	20.6	Less than $9,999	9.2	+11.4
$12,001–24,000	19.9	$10,000–24,999	21.3	−1.4
$24,001–40,000	22.8	$25,000–39,999	18.4	+4.4
More than $40,000	29.9	More than $40,000	51.1	−21.2
Don't know	6.8	—[b]	—	—

Note: Family income level data missing for 1,022 children.

[a]Bureau of the Census (2000a).

[b]U.S. Census does not include a "Don't Know" category.

Establishing Reliability

Internal Consistency   Internal consistency measures the extent to which items on the assessment tool measure the same underlying construct (Salvia & Ysseldyke, 1998). High internal consistency reflects items that assess the same characteristic or behavioral area. To measure internal consistency, coefficient alpha was calculated for each ASQ:SE age interval using the variances of individual items and the variance of the total test scores (N = 1,994). Cronbach's coefficient alphas for the ASQ:SE age intervals are shown in Table A6. Alphas ranged from .67 to .91, with an overall alpha of .82. An alpha of .70 is considered to be an adequate measure of internal consistency (Nunnally, 1978).

Test–Retest Reliability   Test–retest reliability measures the stability of child performance across time. Test–retest reliability for the ASQ:SE was determined by comparing the results of two questionnaires completed by parents at 1- to 3-week intervals. A random sample of parents (N = 367) was asked to complete a second, identical ASQ:SE after returning the first completed questionnaire; parents were "blind"

Table A5.   Number of children by developmental status for ASQ:SE normative sample (N = 2,861)

ASQ:SE age interval	N	Number of subjects by developmental status							
		No risk[a]		At risk[b]		Developmental disability[c]		Social-emotional disability[d]	
		n	Mean	n	Mean	n	Mean	n	Mean
6 month	286	84	19.2	166	20.6	27	29.8	9	77.4
12 month	293	103	22.1	145	26.2	38	40.4	7	67.9
18 month	264	115	22.2	100	32.2	41	68.0	8	97.5
24 month	389	172	25.8	141	37.5	56	46.4	20	86.6
30 month	245	114	33.5	78	46.2	40	86.8	13	107.2
36 month	347	191	33.3	81	47.5	48	81.8	27	119.1
48 month	378	176	31.6	123	52.2	51	76.8	28	130.5
60 month	277	134	30.1	85	47.7	29	69.5	29	132.9
Overall	2,479	1,089	27.2	919	38.8	330	62.4	141	102.4

Note: Developmental status data missing for 382 children.

[a]One or no identified risk factors.

[b]Two or more identified risk factors.

[c]Children receiving early intervention or early childhood special education services.

[d]Children with diagnosed social-emotional disabilities.

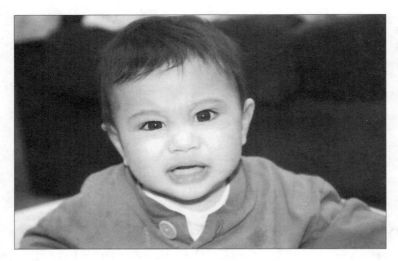

to the results of their first completed ASQ:SE. The percent agreement between classifications of the child's performance on the ASQ:SE at Time 1 (first questionnaire) and Time 2 (second questionnaire) were used to measure test–retest reliability.

Children were classified as "okay" on the ASQ:SE (no further evaluation of social-emotional competence was indicated) if their scores were below the empirically derived cutoff point for that interval. Children were classified as "at risk" on the ASQ:SE (further evaluation of their social-emotional status was indicated) if their scores were on or above the cutoff point. Using the McNemar Test (Agresti, 1990) assessing dependent proportions, test-retest agreement was 94% (*N* = 344/367).

Establishing Validity

The primary goal of a screening measure is to accurately discriminate between individuals who are typical or okay (i.e., do not have the problem or characteristic) on a targeted variable (e.g., development, medical condition such as PKU) and individuals who appear atypical or not okay (i.e., potentially may have the problem or characteristic). Establishing the validity of a screening measure generally requires a two-step process. First, it is necessary to collect sufficient normative data to establish optimal cutoff scores for the screening test. Individuals who fall above the cutoff score are classified as at risk and in need of follow-up, while individuals who score below the cutoff score are classified as okay and do not need follow-up.

Table A6.   Cronbach coefficient alpha by ASQ:SE age interval (*N* = 1,994)

ASQ:SE age interval	Number of questionnaires	Alpha
6 month	196	.69
12 month	196	.67
18 month	210	.81
24 month	297	.80
30 month	198	.88
36 month	281	.89
48 month	317	.91
60 month	299	.91
Overall	1,994	.82

Note: Field-test versions of the B-ASQ (*N* = 867) and Spanish translation (*N* = 153) were not included in this analysis.

For any screening test, there are no absolute scores that separate typical from nontypical individuals. Rather, data must be collected and examined to determine optimal cutoff scores, that is, scores that correctly classify children as needing or not needing follow-up evaluation. Finding optimal cutoff scores requires examining a range of alternatives to discover those scores that maximize the identification of individuals who should receive further testing (i.e., true positives) while minimizing the misidentification of individuals who do not require further testing (i.e., false positives) and minimizing the nonidentification of individuals who should receive further testing (i.e., false negatives).

Once "tentative" cutoff scores are selected, the second step is to determine if they do accurately discriminate between individuals who require follow-up and individuals who do not. Thus, first it is necessary to establish what are thought to be optimal cutoff scores for the screening measure. Once cutoff scores are selected, it is then necessary to determine their accuracy and thus the validity of the screening measure. Establishing the validity of a screening measure is done by comparing an individual's classification on the screening measure with his or her classification on a selected criterion measure(s). Using this two-step process, the validity of the ASQ:SE was examined by comparing children's classification (i.e., developmentally okay or at risk) on the ASQ:SE with their classification (i.e., developmentally okay or at risk/disabled) on selected criterion measures that included the CBCL, the SEEC, and professional diagnosis of a social-emotional disability.

To discover optimal ASQ:SE cutoff scores (i.e., those that yield high true positives, high true negatives, low false positives, and low false negatives), receiver operating characteristic (ROC) curves were used (Swets & Pickett, 1982). ROC analysis permits the systematic comparison of true positive probabilities against false positive probabilities for a range of possible cutoff scores. To create these comparison data, a sample of 1,041 children with completed ASQ:SE questionnaires were given a concurrent criterion measure—either the CBCL or the SEEC—or had a professional diagnosis of a social-emotional disability. Each child's classification (i.e., okay or at risk) on the ASQ:SE was then compared with his or her classification (i.e., okay or at risk/disabled) on one of the criterion measures. Figure 16 in Chapter 5 shows a four-cell contingency table used to assess the agreement between the screening measure (i.e., ASQ:SE) and the follow-up criterion measure (i.e., CBCL, SEEC, or diagnosis of social-emotional disability). In addition, this figure shows the formulas for calculating the percentage of children identified as needing further assessment, percent agreement, sensitivity, specificity, overreferral, underreferral, and positive predictive value.

Comparison of means, medians, interquartile ranges, and ROC cutoffs is shown in Table A7. It can be noted that ROC cutoff scores for most age intervals were similar to scores derived from adding 1.5 semi-interquartile ranges to medians. The general trend of increasingly higher scores as children develop is reflected in both mean and median scores,

Table A7.   Means, medians, interquartile ranges, and ROC by ASQ:SE age interval (N = 2,861)

ASQ:SE age interval	N	Range	Mean	Median	Interquartile range	Median + 1.5 semi-interquartile ranges	ROC cutoff score[a]
6 month	331	0–112.6	22.5	16.7	22.5	34	45
12 month	339	0–145	27.7	25.0	22.0	42	48
18 month	307	0–255	34.6	26.0	26.6	46	50
24 month	441	0–215	35.4	28.4	33.8	54	50
30 month	289	0–290	48.6	35.2	41.5	66	57
36 month	408	0–288	49.9	35.0	48.9	72	59
48 month	447	0–290	55.7	36.0	52.6	75	70
60 month	299	0–293	47.5	35.0	45.0	69	70

Note: Data from the B-ASQ at 6, 12, 24, 30, 36, and 48 months (N = 867) were combined with data from ASQ:SE at the same intervals after *t* tests revealed no significant differences between the field-test version and the ASQ:SE at these age intervals.

[a]ROC cutoff based on "best fit," maximizing true positives and true negatives.

except at 60 months. The leveling or decrease in scores at 60 months may be the artifice of a smaller sample at that age interval.

Frequently, cutoff scores for screening tools are set by using means and standard deviations. That is, the mean score plus one standard deviation is a likely choice for a cutoff score. However, using means to calculate cutoff scores presumes a normal distribution of scores. Score distribution for the ASQ:SE questionnaires was positively skewed—that is, the majority of children obtained low scores (i.e., indicating they have no problem or are okay) and relatively few children obtained high scores (i.e., indicating they have a potential problem or are at risk). Figure A1

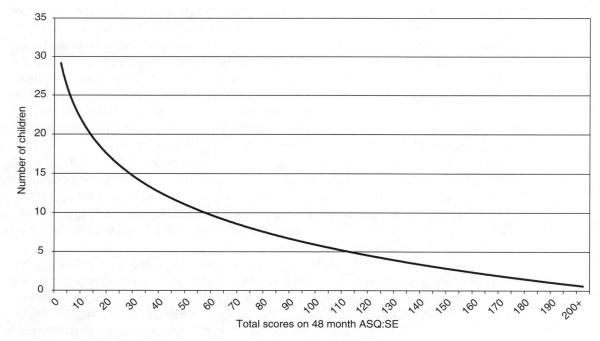

Figure A1.   ASQ:SE total scores by number of children, showing a positively skewed distribution.

shows the positively skewed distribution of scores for the 48 month ASQ:SE; other age intervals showed similar score distributions. Means and standard deviations were not used for determining cutoff points because of the positive skew of ASQ:SE scores across intervals. Instead, ROC analyses were conducted to determine the best cutoff point for each interval.

To examine gender differences, scores for males and females were compared. Mean and median scores by gender are presented in Table A8. Box plots were then derived to examine the score distributions by gender. Box plots for the 30 and 36 month ASQ:SE male and female score distributions are shown in Figure A2. Box plots provide a visual "picture" of a distribution. The bottom line of the box is the 25th percentile, or Quartile 1. The top line of the box is the 75th percentile, or Quartile 3. The middle line is the median, or Quartile 2; the mean is indicated by the +. Whiskers (lines) extend to the highest and lowest observations, but not further than 1.5 interquartile ranges from the median. Outliers beyond 1.5 interquartile ranges are indicated by O; outliers beyond 3 interquartile ranges are indicated by O*.

As shown in Figure A2, the majority of scores for males at the 30 month interval range between 25 and 75, with the 1.5 interquartile range extending to 0 and to 160. Outliers extend upward to 300. For females, the range is between 20 and 50, with the 1.5 interquartile range extending to 75. Outliers extend beyond 200. A similar distribution for both males and females can be seen at the 36 month interval. Similar distribution patterns occurred at all age intervals and indicate, in general, that males tend to have greater dispersal of scores and more extreme scores.

When gender group differences are compared using the nonparametric Kruskal-Wallis Test (Heiman, 1992), significant differences are found at 30, 36, 48, and 60 months, as shown in Table A8. It is important to note that the validity sample currently does not have adequate numbers of females with social-emotional problems to indicate whether separate cutoff scores for females are needed. Consequently, girls whose scores are close to the cutoffs at the 30, 36, 48, and 60 month intervals should be considered for referral. As additional data are added to the validity sample, revised cutoffs, if necessary, will be posted on the Paul H. Brookes Publishing Co. website (http://www.brookespublishing.com).

MODIFYING CUTOFF SCORES

If programs want to modify cutoff scores, semi-interquartile ranges (i.e., median + [quartile 1 – quartile 3] / 2) should be used as the basis for modification. See the Paul H. Brookes Publishing Co. website (http://www.brookespublishing.com/asqse) for discussion of guidelines for altering ASQ:SE cutoff points.

Table A8.   ASQ:SE mean and median scores for males and females by age interval (N = 2,801)

ASQ:SE age interval	Male (N = 1,421)			Female (N = 1,380)		
	N	Mean	Median	N	Mean	Median
6 month	164	25.4	20.0	163	20.5	15.0
12 month	171	27.7	25.0	163	27.0	25.0
18 month	140	37.7	25.0	164	33.2	30.0
24 month	233	39.1	31.2	205	32.5	25.0
30 month	163	57.3	37.6	123	39.1***	33.4
36 month	190	58.3	40.0	200	40.4***	30.0
48 month	212	61.8	46.4	214	40.3***	26.6
60 month	148	57.8	40.6	148	36.4***	25.0

Note: Gender data missing for 60 children.

***Significant at $p < .001$.

Once optimal cutoff scores were established, the next step was to examine the agreement between the classification of children using these cutoffs with selected criterion measures. Both concurrent and known groups validity of the ASQ:SE have been examined, and the findings are reported in the following two sections.

Examining Concurrent Validity

To determine how accurately the ASQ:SE discriminates between children whose social-emotional development is proceeding without problem and children who have or who are at risk for developing social-emotional problems, a comparison with selected criterion measures was necessary. Criterion measures chosen to examine the concurrent validity, or discriminative power, of the ASQ:SE were the CBCL and SEEC.

The CBCL is a well-studied tool with reported adequate psychometric properties (Achenbach, 1991, 1992) and is consider the "gold standard" against which most new tools assessing social-emotional competence are measured (McConaughy, 1992). The CBCL has two forms, one for ages 2–3 years (CBCL/2-3; Achenbach, 1992) and one for ages 4–18 years (CBCL/4-18; Achenbach, 1991). Children who had scores of 61 or above on the CBCL/2-3 and of 64 or above on the CBCL/4-18 were classified as having social-emotional disabilities. (Achenbach & Rescorla's CBCL/1½–5 was not published until 2000; a decision was made to retain the CBCL/2-3 for all ASQ:SE psychometric studies.)

The SEEC is a measure frequently used to assess the social-emotional competence of young children. Psychometric data on the SEEC suggest it is both reliable and valid (Sparrow et al., 1998), although new studies have not been conducted since the original study of the Vineland Adaptive Behavior Scale (Sparrow, Balla, & Cicchetti, 1984) in the 1980s. While the CBCL was completed by parents or caregivers in their homes, the SEEC was completed through an interview with the parent. Children were classified as having a social-emotional disability if their scores on the SEEC were 70 or below (Sparrow et al., 1998).

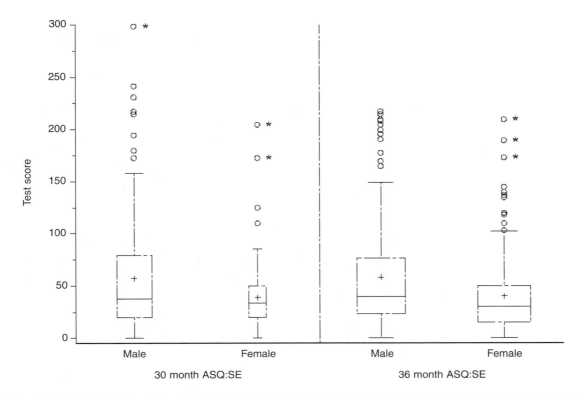

Figure A2. Box plots for 30 and 36 month ASQ:SE by gender. Box plots illustrate the distribution of scores. Bottom line of box is 25th percentile, or Quartile 1. Top line of box is 75th percentile, or Quartile 3. Middle line of box is the median, or Quartile 2. Mean is indicted by +. Whiskers (lines) extend to the highest and lowest observations, but not further than 1.5 interquartile ranges. Outliers beyond 1.5 interquartile ranges are indicated by **O**. Outliers beyond 3 interquartile ranges are indicated by **O***. Box width varies with *n*.

Parents or other primary caregivers of children in the validity sample (*N* = 1,041) completed either the CBLC or the SEEC within 2–3 weeks of completing the ASQ:SE on their child. In addition, the validity sample included 88 children ranging in age from 2½ to 5 years who had been professionally diagnosed as having a social-emotional disability and were receiving intervention services. Parents completed an ASQ:SE on these children as well.

Children in the validity sample were classified as either okay or at risk based on their ASQ:SE scores and the established cutoffs and were independently classified as either okay or at risk/disabled using their scores on the CBLC or SEEC or based on professional diagnosis. These two independent classifications were then compared for all children in the validity sample. One of four outcomes was possible: 1) the ASQ:SE and criterion measure both classified the child as okay (i.e., true negatives); 2) the ASQ:SE and criterion measure both classified the child as at risk/disabled (i.e., true positives); 3) the ASQ:SE classified the child as okay, while the criterion measure classified the child as at risk/disabled (i.e., false negatives); and 4) the ASQ:SE classified the child as at risk while the criterion measure classified the child as okay (i.e., false positives).

To conduct these comparisons, contingency tables containing four cells (i.e., A = true positives, B = false positives, C = false negatives, and D = true negatives, as shown in Figure 16 in Chapter 5) were developed for each of the ASQ:SE age intervals using the ROC cutoff scores listed in Table A7. Each contingency table contained in Figure A3 shows the absolute agreement for true positives, false positives, false negatives, and true negatives. From the data contained in the contingency table, the sensitivity, specificity, false positive rate, true positive rate, false negative rate, percent agreement, underreferral, overreferral, percent referral, and positive predictive value were calculated for each ASQ:SE age interval. An overall comparison across all intervals is shown in Figure A4.

Table A9 presents a comparison of the sensitivity, specificity, false positive rate, false negative rate, percent agreement, underreferral, and overreferral across ASQ:SE age intervals. Sensitivity ranged from a low of 70.8% at 24 months to a high of 84.6% at 60 months. Specificity ranged from 89.5% at 30 months to 98.2% at 6 months. Percent agreement ranged from 87.8% at 30 months to 94.0% at 60 months. Underreferral ranged from 2.4% at 60 months to 4.7% at 12 months, while overreferral ranged from 3.0% at 18 months to 8.6% at 30 months. These findings suggest the ASQ:SE is generally accurate in discriminating between children who are developing okay and those who need follow-up. In practical terms, the underreferral rate appears acceptable across intervals and never exceeds 4.6%, while the false positive and overreferral rate are consistently high. This finding suggests that parents using the ASQ:SE are consistently identifying problems in their children that the criterion measures do not. At least two possible explanations seem reasonable. First, the ASQ:SE may be consistently overscreening children, or second, the criterion measures may consistently be missing children who have social-emotional problems. Only follow-up of overreferred children (using the criterion measure classification) will determine which explanation is correct.

Examining Known Groups Validity

Another approach to assessing validity of a screening measure suggested by Spector (1992) requires examining the differences in scores across groups. For this analysis, children in the validity sample were divided into four groups based on their developmental risk status: no risk, at risk, developmental disability, and social-emotional disability. Children were assigned to the no-risk group if parents reported one or no risk factors (N = 812), were assigned to the at-risk group if parents reported two or more risk factors (N = 790), were assigned to the developmental disability group if they were receiving general early intervention services (N = 297), or were assigned to the social-emotional disability group if they had been diagnosed with a behavior or emotional problem and were receiving intervention services (N = 88). Risk factors included 1) annual family income less than $12,000; 2) mother less than 18 years old when child was born; 3) mother's level of education less than high school graduation; 4) in-

6 month ASQ:SE

		Criterion measure classification		
		At risk	*Okay*	
ASQ:SE	*At risk*	11	1	12
classification	*Okay*	3	56	59
	Total	14	57	71

Sensitivity	Specificity	False positive	True positive	False negative	Percent agreement	Under-referral	Over-referral	Percent referral	Positive predictive value
78.6%	98.2%	8.3%	78.6%	5.1%	94.0%	4.2%	1.4%	17.0%	91%

12 month ASQ:SE

		Criterion measure classification		
		At risk	*Okay*	
ASQ:SE	*At risk*	10	2	12
classification	*Okay*	4	69	73
	Total	14	71	85

Sensitivity	Specificity	False positive	True positive	False negative	Percent agreement	Under-referral	Over-referral	Percent referral	Positive predictive value
71.4%	97.2%	16.7%	71.4%	5.5%	93.0%	4.7%	2.4%	15.0%	83%

18 month ASQ:SE

		Criterion measure classification		
		At risk	*Okay*	
ASQ:SE	*At risk*	9	3	12
classification	*Okay*	3	84	87
	Total	12	87	99

Sensitivity	Specificity	False positive	True positive	False negative	Percent agreement	Under-referral	Over-referral	Percent referral	Positive predictive value
75.0%	96.6%	25.0%	75.0%	3.4%	93.9%	3.0%	3.0%	12.0%	75%

24 month ASQ:SE

		Criterion measure classification		
		At risk	*Okay*	
ASQ:SE	*At risk*	17	9	26
classification	*Okay*	7	119	126
	Total	24	128	152

Sensitivity	Specificity	False positive	True positive	False negative	Percent agreement	Under-referral	Over-referral	Percent referral	Positive predictive value
70.8%	93.0%	34.6%	70.8%	5.6%	89.5%	4.6%	5.9%	17.0%	65%

(continued)

Figure A3. Contingency tables showing agreement between ASQ:SE classification and criterion measure classification and ASQ:SE sensitivity, specificity, false positive rate, true positive rate, false negative rate, percent agreement, underreferral, overreferral, percent referral, and positive predictive value by age interval (definitions and formulas are contained in Figure 16 in Chapter 5). Criterion measure classification includes CBCL, SEEC, and professional diagnosis.

Figure A3. *(continued)*

30 month ASQ:SE

		Criterion measure classification		
		At risk	*Okay*	
ASQ:SE	*At risk*	10	19	29
classification	*Okay*	3	84	87
	Total	13	103	116

Sensitivity	Specificity	False positive	True positive	False negative	Percent agreement	Under-referral	Over-referral	Percent referral	Positive predictive value
80.0%	89.5%	38.5%	80.0%	4.5%	87.8%	3.4%	8.6%	23.0%	61%

36 month ASQ:SE

		Criterion measure classification		
		At risk	*Okay*	
ASQ:SE	*At risk*	28	10	38
classification	*Okay*	8	133	141
	Total	36	143	179

Sensitivity	Specificity	False positive	True positive	False negative	Percent agreement	Under-referral	Over-referral	Percent referral	Positive predictive value
77.8%	93.0%	26.3%	77.8%	5.7%	89.9%	4.5%	5.7%	21.0%	73%

48 month ASQ:SE

		Criterion measure classification		
		At risk	*Okay*	
ASQ:SE	*At risk*	20	8	28
classification	*Okay*	6	140	146
	Total	26	148	174

Sensitivity	Specificity	False positive	True positive	False negative	Percent agreement	Under-referral	Over-referral	Percent referral	Positive predictive value
76.9%	94.6%	28.6%	76.9%	4.1%	92.0%	3.4%	4.6%	16.0%	71%

60 month ASQ:SE

		Criterion measure classification		
		At risk	*Okay*	
ASQ:SE	*At risk*	22	6	28
classification	*Okay*	4	136	140
	Total	26	142	168

Sensitivity	Specificity	False positive	True positive	False negative	Percent agreement	Under-referral	Over-referral	Percent referral	Positive predictive value
84.6%	95.8%	21.4%	84.6%	2.9%	94.0%	2.4%	3.6%	18.1%	71%

Overall

		Criterion measure classification			
		At risk	*Okay*		
ASQ:SE	*At risk*	131	48	179	
classification	*Okay*	37	825	862	
	Total	168	873	1,041	

Sensitivity	Specificity	False positive	True positive	False negative	Percent agreement	Under-referral	Over-referral	Percent referral	Positive predictive value
78.0%	94.5%	26.8%	78.0%	4.3%	91.8%	3.6%	4.6%	17.2%	26.8%

Figure A4. Contingency table showing overall agreement (combined across age intervals) between ASQ:SE classification and criterion measure classification and ASQ:SE sensitivity, specificity, false positive rate, true positive rate, false negative rate, percent agreement, underreferral, overreferral, percent referral, and positive predictive value by age interval (definitions and formulas are contained in Figure 16 in Chapter 5). Criterion measure classification includes CBCL, SEEC, and professional diagnosis.

volvement of child protective services with family; 5) child in foster care; and 6) birth weight less than 3 pounds, 5 ounces.

Figure A5 presents the mean scores for the four groups across the 6, 12, 18, 24, 30, 36, 48, and 60 month ASQ:SE intervals. Differences between risk groups were examined using the nonparametric Kruskal-Wallis Test (Heiman, 1992). Significant differences (p < .0001) were found between groups at all ASQ:SE age intervals. These findings suggest the ASQ:SE can accurately discriminate between children whose social-emotional development is typical and those who have disabilities. An example of box plots showing the distribution of risk groups for the 48 month ASQ:SE is presented in Figure A6. The box plots clearly show that mean (marked with +) and median (middle horizontal line in each box) scores increase as risk factors increase. In addition, there is almost no overlap in the distribution of scores between the no risk and social-emotional disability groups. Children with diagnosed social-emotional disabilities had the highest scores, while children in the no risk group had the lowest scores.

Table A9.   ASQ:SE cutoff scores and classification statistics by age interval based on ROC cutoff score (*N* = 1,041)

ASQ:SE age interval	N	Cutoff score	Sensitivity	Specificity	False positive rate	False negative rate	Percent agreement	Under-referral	Over-referral
6 month	71	45	78.6	98.2	8.3	5.1	94.0	4.2	1.4
12 month	85	48	71.4	97.2	16.7	5.5	93.0	4.7	2.4
18 month	99	50	75.0	96.6	25.0	3.4	93.9	3.0	3.0
24 month	152	50	70.8	93.0	34.6	5.6	89.5	4.6	5.9
30 month	115	57	80.0	89.5	38.5	4.5	87.8	3.4	8.6
36 month	179	59	77.8	93.0	26.3	5.7	89.9	4.5	5.7
48 month	174	70	76.9	94.6	28.6	4.1	92.0	3.4	4.6
60 month	168	70	84.6	95.8	21.4	2.9	94.0	2.4	3.6
Overall	1,041		78.0	94.5	26.8	4.3	91.8	3.6	4.6

Note: See Figure 16 in Chapter 5 for formulas used in calculating classification statistics.

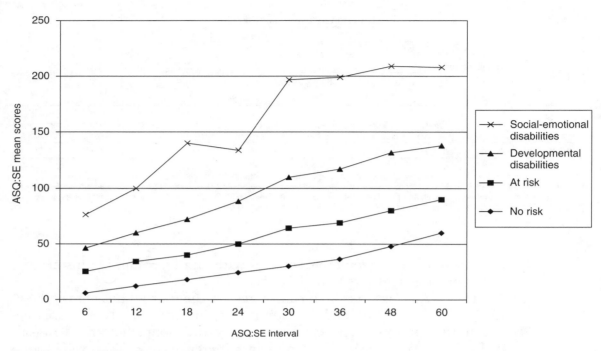

Figure A5.   Mean ASQ:SE scores by group risk status.

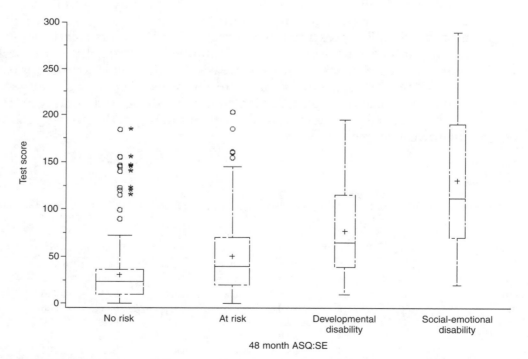

Figure A6.   Box plots of distribution of total scores on 48 month ASQ:SE by developmental status. Box plots illustrate the spread of distribution. Bottom line of box is 25th percentile, or Quartile 1. Top line of box is 75th percentile, or Quartile 3. Middle line of box is the median, or Quartile 2. Mean is indicted by +. Whiskers (lines) extend to the highest and lowest observations, but not further than 1.5 interquartile ranges. Outliers beyond 1.5 interquartile ranges are indicated by **O**. Outliers beyond 3 interquartile ranges are indicated by **O***. Box width varies with *n*.

UTILITY STUDIES

Utility of a screening tool measures the usefulness or practicality of the test or procedure (Bricker & Squires, 1989). A random sample of parents (N = 731) who completed the ASQ:SE were asked to complete a utility questionnaire that requested their opinion about the length, appropriateness, and ease of completion of the ASQ:SE. Summary results of the utility questionnaire can be found in Table A10. Sixty percent of the respondents indicated that it took less than 10 minutes to complete. Ninety-six percent of the respondents indicated the ASQ:SE was easy to understand; ninety percent noted that question content was appropriate. Thus, parents reported that the ASQ:SE was easy to understand, that it took little time to complete, and that the questions were appropriate.

In addition, parents indicated that completing the ASQ:SE was interesting and helped them to think about the social and emotional development of their young children. Six parents thought that questions related to sexual interest on the 36, 48, and 60 month ASQ:SE were inappropri-

Table A10.   Parent responses (N = 731) to ASQ:SE utility questionnaire items

Question	Percentage of parents reporting
1. How long to complete ASQ:SE?	(Missing 4 responses)
a. Less than 10 minutes	60
b. 10–20 minutes	32
c. 20–30 minutes	4
d. 30 minutes–1 hour	0
e. More than 1 hour	0
2. Was ASQ:SE easy to understand?	(Missing 7 responses)
a. Yes	96
b. Sometimes	3
c. No	0
3. Were ASQ:SE questions appropriate?	(Missing 13 responses)
a. Yes	90
b. Sometimes	7
c. No	1
4. The ASQ:SE questionnaire was . . . (check all that apply)	
a. Fun to do	38
b. Interesting	57
c. Took too long	1
d. Helped me think about my child	71
e. Waste of time	2
f. Didn't tell me much	10
5. Would you fill out another ASQ:SE?	(Missing 33 responses)
a. Yes	91
b. No	5
6. Would you change the ASQ:SE?	
a. Yes	16
b. No	84

ate; however, a decision was made to retain these items because of their importance to identification of disturbances related to sexual abuse and early exposure to domestic violence.

SUMMARY

Psychometric studies on the ASQ:SE are summarized in this Technical Report. Normative data were based on 3,014 completed questionnaires; validity studies were conducted using 1,041 children. Internal consistency measured by coefficient alpha was found to be high across intervals, ranging from .67 to .91 with an overall alpha of .82. Test–retest reliability, measured as the agreement between two ASQ:SE questionnaires completed by parents at 1- to 3-week intervals was 94%. Sensitivity ranged from 71% at 24 months to 85% at 60 months, with 78% overall sensitivity. Specificity of the questionnaires ranged from 90% at 30 months to 98% at 6 months, with 94% overall. Percent agreement between questionnaires and standardized assessments/disability status ranged from 88% at 30 months to 94% at 60 months, with overall agreement of 92%. Underreferral ranged from 2.4% at 60 months to 4.7% at 12 months, while overreferral ranged from 3.0% at 18 months to 8.6% at 30 months. The ability of the ASQ:SE to detect atypical social-emotional development (sensitivity) was generally lower across intervals, while specificity, or the ability of the ASQ:SE to correctly identify typically developing children, was high. Specificity may have been elevated in the 6, 12, and 18 month intervals because of the large number of "identified" children in these samples and the small number of low-moderate risk children.

Research is continuing on the ASQ:SE. Specifically, additional young children with atypical social-emotional development—particularly girls—are being recruited for validity studies. In addition, results of ASQ:SE completed by parents and teachers are being compared to study its interrater reliability. Research findings will be posted at the Paul H. Brookes Publishing Co. website (http://www.brookespublishing.com) as they become available.

REFERENCES

Achenbach, T. (1991). *Manual for the Child Behavior Checklist/4–18 and 1991 profile.* Burlington: University of Vermont, Department of Psychiatry.

Achenbach, T. (1992). *Manual for the Child Behavior Checklist/2–3 and 1992 profile.* Burlington: University of Vermont, Department of Psychiatry.

Achenbach, T., & Rescorla, L. (2000). *Manual for the ASEBA preschool forms and profiles.* Burlington, VT: ASEBA.

Agresti, A. (1990). *Categorical data analysis.* New York: John Wiley & Sons.

American Psychiatric Association. (1994). *Diagnostic and statistical manual of mental disorders* (4th ed.). Washington, DC: Author.

Bricker, D., & Squires, J. (1989). The effectiveness of screening at-risk infants: Infant Monitoring Questionnaire. *Topics in Early Special Childhood Education, 3*(9), 67–85.

Bureau of the Census. (2000a, September). *Table 13. Money income in the United States: Current population reports: Consumer income, 1999, P60-209* [On-line]. Available: http://www.census.gov.

Bureau of the Census. (2000b, December). *Table 1: Educational attainment of the population 15 years and over, by sex (female, all races)* [On-line]. Available: http://www.census.gov.

Bureau of the Census. (2001, April). *PHC-T-1: Population by race and Hispanic or Latino origin* [On-line]. Available: http://www.census.gov.

Filipek, P.A., Accardo, P.J., Ashwall, S., et al. (2000). Practice parameter. Screening and diagnosis of autism: Report of the Quality Standards Subcommittee of the American Academy of Neurology and the Child Neurology Society. *Neurology, 55*(4), 468–479.

Filipek, P.A., Accardo, P.J., Baranek, G.T., et al. (1999). The screening and diagnosis of autistic spectrum disorders. *Journal of Autism and Developmental Disorders, 29*(6), 439–484.

Heiman, G. (1992). *Basic statistics for the behavioral sciences.* Boston: Houghton Mifflin.

McConaughy, S.H. (1992). Objective assessment of children's behavioral and emotional problems. In C.E. Walker & M.C. Roberts (Eds.), *Handbook of clinical child psychology* (pp. 163–180). New York: John Wiley & Sons.

Nunnally, J.C. (1978). *Psychometric theory* (2nd ed.). New York, McGraw-Hill.

Salvia, J., & Ysseldyke, J. (1998). *Assessment* (7th ed.). Boston: Houghton Mifflin.

Sparrow, S., Balla, D., & Cicchetti, D. (1984). *Vineland Adaptive Behavior Scales (VABS).* Circle Pines, MN: American Guidance Service.

Sparrow, S., Balla, D., & Cicchetti, D. (1998). *Vineland Social-Emotional Early Childhood Scale (SEEC).* Circle Pines, MN: American Guidance Service.

Spector, P. (1992). *Summated rating scale construction.* Newbury Park, NJ: Sage University Press.

Squires, J., Bricker, D., Twombly, E., Yockelson, S., & Kim, Y. (1996). *Behavior-Ages & Stages Questionnaires.* Eugene: University of Oregon, Center on Human Development.

Swets, J.A., & Pickett, R.M. (1982). *Evaluation of diagnostic systems: Methods from signal detection theory.* San Diego: Academic Press.

B

ASQ:SE Supplemental Forms and Procedures

ASQ:SE

Suggested steps to take when establishing a monitoring program using the ASQ:SE are described in this appendix. Specifically, steps to assemble a child file and a suggested demographic form are given. Management options including developing a card file tickler system for the questionnaires are explained. Procedures for questionnaire mail-out, interviewing, and home visiting are described in detail, and sample forms are included.

ASSEMBLING THE CHILD FILE

Assembling individual files for each participant ensures that all questionnaires and forms concerning the family and the child's progress will be kept in a central location so that, when necessary, information can be obtained efficiently. For example, forms such as the Child and Family Demographic Information Form, shown in Figure B1, should be kept in the front of the file because they may be needed frequently. All of the information in the file should be checked and/or updated periodically.

Developing a child file is best accomplished by completing the following steps:

1. Assign the child ID number. The first child to join the program might be assigned the number 001, the second 002, and so forth. ID numbers should be assigned for two reasons. First, children with the same or similar last names are less likely to be confused if ID numbers are assigned. Second, the use of ID numbers can ensure confidentiality when necessary.

2. Place the Child and Family Demographic Information Form at the front of the file. If for some reason the information on this form has not been collected, it should be obtained before proceeding.

3. Complete a Child Information Summary Form, on which are recorded basic identifying data (see Figure B2). Add this form to the child file.

Joanna Blanding is the director of a program called Good Start. Good Start is a home visiting program that serves young mothers, providing them with support, information about their new babies, and links to community services. Joanna and her staff have decided to use the ASQ:SE in their work with families and have started to develop a system within their organization. The program already assigns children an identification (ID) number and collects demographic information, and staff recently created a form similar to the ASQ:SE Master List Form to make sure all of the families and primary health care providers were informed and had provided consent to participate in the screening project. Joanna has prepared the master set of the ASQ:SE questionnaires and added the agency's logo and contact information on the forms. She has designated a support staff person to make copies of the questionnaires and notify her about which children will require screening activities each month. The support staff has created and managed a card file tickler system that will notify her of upcoming screening activities, and she in turn has notified home visitors and supplied them with materials (i.e., ASQ:SE questionnaires and Information Summary forms). Home visitors have been given a mini-training about how to introduce the ASQ:SE to families and were given a copy of the ASQ:SE Home Visiting Procedures outlined on pp. 108–110 of this appendix. The home visitors are responsible for gathering information from parents, scoring questionnaires, and responding to families' interests and concerns. Staff meetings, at which questionable scores and referrals were discussed, will be held on a biweekly basis, providing structure, support, and information for home visitors regarding the results of the ASQ:SE.

4. Record the child's age. The ASQ:SE does not use "corrected age" for a child born prematurely; however, corrected age may be used for up to 24 months of age if an agency is already correcting a baby's age for prematurity.

5. Enter the child's name and ID number on the program's ASQ:SE Master List Form. Figure B3 is a blank ASQ:SE Master List Form that may be photocopied and modified to meet the needs of specific programs. This list of participating children is essential to the smooth and efficient operation of a screening and monitoring system because it assists program personnel in ensuring that necessary information is collected and questionnaires are completed.

6. Label the file with the child's name, ID number, and other information that program personnel may find essential (e.g., date of birth).

7. Store the file in an accessible but secure location.

Child and Family Demographic Information Form

ASQ:SE

1. ID # _____
2. Child's name _____
   Parent's or guardian's name (last, first) _____
3. Address: Number, street _____
   Town/City _____
   County _____ State/Province _____ ZIP/Postal code _____
   Telephone: Home _____
   Work _____
4. Child's date of birth (month/day/year) _____ / _____ / _____
5. Child's sex (male/female) _____
6. Ethnicity of child _____
7. Child's birth weight (in pounds/ounces) _____
8. In neonatal intensive care unit? (yes/no) _____
   Length of time (in days) _____
9. Date of admission to monitoring program (month/day/year) _____ / _____ / _____
10. Child status:
    At risk? (yes/no) _____
    If yes, list three primary risk factors: _____
    Disability?(yes/no) _____ Disability (list) _____
11. Is this an adoptive family? (yes/no) _____ or a foster family? _____
12. Age of biological mother (in years) _____
13. Mother's birth surname _____
14. Mother's marital status _____
15. Highest level of education of mother _____
16. Highest level of education of partner _____
17. Occupation of mother _____
18. Occupation of partner _____
19. Estimated yearly household income _____
20. Physician _____
    Telephone (or name of clinic) _____
21. Has child had any medical or developmental problems? (yes/no) _____
    If yes, explain _____
22. Total number of children in household _____

The ASQ:SE User's Guide, Squires, Bricker, and Twombly. © 2002 Paul H. Brookes Publishing Co.

Figure B1.   A sample Child and Family Demographic Information Form. This form or one like it should be easily accessible throughout the child's involvement in the program. A Spanish translation of this form is provided in Appendix G.

CREATING A CARD FILE TICKLER SYSTEM

When monitoring groups of children, a system must be created to alert program staff as to when activities (e.g., filling out a questionnaire, calling families to have questionnaires returned) should occur. A simple and inexpensive way is to create a card file tickler box, discussed next, although many programs may choose to develop their own system or utilize computer based systems.

To begin, locate a 5" × 8" index card (or other size) file box. Place dividers for each month (e.g., January, February, March), with weekly sub-

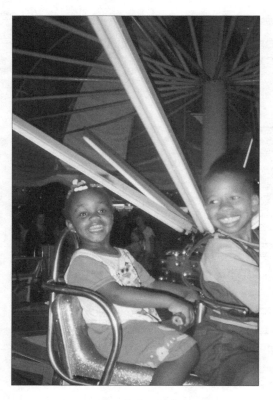

dividers included for each month, in the file box. Programs may choose to arrange the subdividers by day, week, fortnight, or month, depending on the number of children monitored. Complete an individual index card for each child monitored in the program. Figure B4 shows a sample card for a child named Ramal Jones. A blank sample card is provided in Figure B5 for program staff to photocopy on an as-needed basis. The card contains space to record essential identifying information for the child and family, as well as a tracking grid to assist program staff.

The tracking grid includes a column listing the program's planned activities in the order they are to be administered and columns for each age interval at which a questionnaire is to be completed. Upon completion of each activity in the first column, staff enter the date in the appropriate column. The activities column contains entries for follow-up, which may not be necessary if the questionnaire is completed and returned to the program on schedule. After a questionnaire is mailed or given to the parents, the card is refiled in chronological order according to the month and week the ques-

---

ID # _____   **ASQ:SE**

Child Information Summary Form

1. Child's name _____
2. Child's date of birth (month/day/year) _____ / _____ / _____
3. Sex (male/female) _____
4. Parent or guardian's name (last, first) _____
5. Other caregiver(s) _____
6. Address: Number, street _____
        Town/City _____
        County _____ State/Province _____ ZIP/Postal Code _____
   Telephone: Home _____
           Work _____
7. Primary health care provider _____
   Telephone (or name of clinic) _____
8. Notes/comments _____
   _____
   _____

The ASQ:SE User's Guide, Squires, Bricker, and Twombly. © 2002 Paul H. Brookes Publishing Co.

Figure B2.   The Child Information Summary Form should be completed during the first step of the implementation phase. It should be kept in the child's file. A Spanish translation of this form is provided in Appendix G.

ASQ:SE Master List Form

Site _____

Child's name	ID#	Parent consent	Child and Family Demographic Info. Form	Physician info. letter	Child Information Summary Form	Child file card	6 month ASQ:SE	12 month ASQ:SE	18 month ASQ:SE	24 month ASQ:SE	30 month ASQ:SE	36 month ASQ:SE	48 month ASQ:SE	60 month ASQ:SE

The ASQ:SE User's Guide, Squires, Bricker, and Twombly. © 2002 Paul H. Brookes Publishing Co.

Figure B3.   Program staff should be diligent in keeping the ASQ:SE Master List Form up to date. Every child who is participating in the program should be listed by name and ID number on this form or one like it.

Child's name _Ramal Jones_
Parent's or guardian's name _Frieda Jones_
Address _Chicago, IL_
Telephone _555-2707_

Child's sex _M_
Date of birth _Sept. 30, 2000_
Message telephone/address _None_

ACTIVITIES	6 month	12 month	18 month	24 month	30 month	36 month	48 month	60 month
Send questionnaire		9-23-01		9/23/02				
Sent questionnaire		9-23-01						
Call—instructions		9-26-01						
Called		9-26-01						
Expected return		10-7-01						
Returned		10-7-01						
If not returned, called								
Results		OK						
Feedback sent		10-10-01						
Parent called with concern		—						
Physician notified		—						
Referral		—						
Refile card (y/n)		Y						
Comments								

The ASQ:SE User's Guide, Squires, Bricker, and Twombly. © 2002 Paul H. Brookes Publishing Co.

Figure B4. The card file tickler system includes a card for each child participating in the program. As shown on this sample card completed for Ramal Jones, essential identifying information is recorded and staff use the grid to track the distribution and return of questionnaires. Basic results are also recorded. *Message telephone/address* provides a space to record an alternate contact in case the family moves between questionnaire intervals. The blank card in Figure B5 may be photocopied for program use.

Child's name _____
Parent's or guardian's name _____
Address _____
Telephone _____

Child's sex _____
Date of birth _____
Message telephone/address _____

ACTIVITIES	6 month	12 month	18 month	24 month	30 month	36 month	48 month	60 month
Send questionnaire								
Sent questionnaire								
Call—instructions								
Called								
Expected return								
Returned								
If not returned, called								
Results								
Feedback sent								
Parent called with concern								
Physician notified								
Referral								
Refile card (y/n)								
Comments								

Figure B5.   A blank tickler file card.

The ASQ:SE User's Guide, Squires, Bricker, and Twombly. © 2002 Paul H. Brookes Publishing Co.

tionnaire should be returned. All activities associated with tracking the child's progress are filed by date under the appropriate month and week.

The card file tickler system includes a card for each child participating in the program. As shown on the sample card in Figure B4 completed for Ramal Jones, essential identifying information is recorded, and staff use the grid to track the distribution and return of questionnaires. Basic results are also recorded.

For example, Ramal's card is filed under the week of September 26 because that date is approximately 1 week before Ramal will become 12 months old. When September 23 arrives, the card is reviewed, and Ramal's mother is sent a 12 month ASQ:SE questionnaire. A notation is made on the card indicating that a reminder call should be made to the mother on September 30, or approximately 3–5 days after the questionnaire was mailed, and that the questionnaire should be returned by October 7. The card is filed under the week of September 30 until the call is made and the questionnaire is returned.

If the questionnaire arrives before October 7, this is indicated on the card. In addition, other important information should be recorded on the card when possible (e.g., feedback sent, results of questionnaire, whether child was referred for services). A space is also provided at the bottom of the card to record any additional comments or information relevant to the child. The date for mailing the next questionnaire is recorded, and the card is refiled under the appropriate month and day.

Ramal's mother returned the questionnaire on October 7; the results indicated typical social-emotional development, and staff sent feedback to Ms. Jones on October 10. If Ramal's mother had not returned the questionnaire by October 7, a staff member would have called her, and a new expected return date would have been recorded with the card being filed under this new date.

Specific steps for following this card file tickler system are outlined next. In all steps, *target* refers to the assigned date for completing the questionnaire.

1. Enter the child's name and additional identifying information at the top of the card.
2. Enter the target date minus 1–2 weeks under the appropriate age interval column to indicate when the questionnaire should be mailed or given to the parents or service providers who will be completing the form. File the card in the box under that date.
3. Mail or give the questionnaire to the parents or service provider 1–2 weeks before the target date. Record the date the questionnaire is mailed or given to whomever will be completing it. Do not include the ASQ:SE Information Summary if mailing the questionnaire to a parent.
4. If program resources permit, plan to call the parents or service provider completing the questionnaire 1 or 2 days before the target

date. File the card under the date when this call should be made. During this telephone call, answer any questions and encourage prompt return of the questionnaire. Record the date of this conversation on the child's file card. Calculate the expected date of return, which is the target date plus 1–2 weeks, and enter this date on the card. Refile the child's card under the target date.

5. If the questionnaire is returned on or before the expected return date, record the date it is received.

6. If the questionnaire has not been returned by the expected return date, call the parent or service provider who agreed to complete the questionnaire. If resources permit, call again 3 or 4 days later if the questionnaire still has not been returned. If the parents cannot be reached by telephone, send a reminder and/or duplicate questionnaire in the mail. If the parents cannot be contacted by any means, make a note of this and the reasons (e.g., telephone disconnected).

7. Once completed, the questionnaire should be scored and appropriate next steps taken according to the ASQ:SE Referral Criteria outlined in Chapter 4 of this *User's Guide.*

8. Send a feedback letter and ASQ:SE activities and developmental guide (see Appendix C) if resources permit.

9. If a referral must be made, note the date on the child's file card and proceed accordingly.

10. If a referral is not made, file the card under the next target date.

MAIL-OUT PROCEDURES

The ASQ:SE system can be used in a mail-out format. This system fits the needs of programs that screen children whose parents are capable of reading, observing and indicating their children's behaviors, and mailing back the questionnaires.

In each master set of questionnaires, a master mail-out and mail-back sheet is provided. (An example is shown in Figure B6.) For programs that decide to use this format, the name of the screening program and its address should be stamped, printed, or typed on the mail-back (bottom) portion; and the parent's name and address should be written or typed on the mail-out (top) portion. A contact person should be identified who can answer any questions or concerns parents may have while completing the questionnaire. Once the identifying information for the child is completed and the questionnaire is ready to be mailed out, the questionnaire may be stapled or taped at the ends and top. A stamp for return postage should be included, to increase the return rate. Staff may prefer to use an envelope to mail the questionnaires; in these cases, a stamped, addressed return envelope should also be enclosed to encourage return of the completed questionnaires.

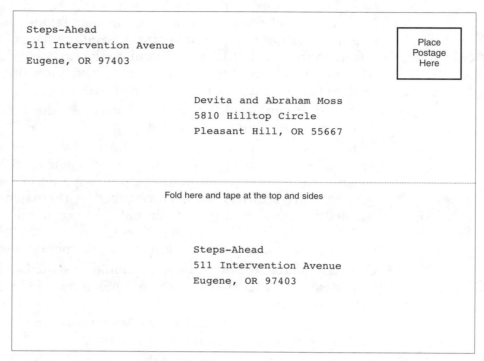

Steps-Ahead
511 Intervention Avenue
Eugene, OR 97403

Place
Postage
Here

Devita and Abraham Moss
5810 Hilltop Circle
Pleasant Hill, OR 55667

Fold here and tape at the top and sides

Steps-Ahead
511 Intervention Avenue
Eugene, OR 97403

The ASQ:SE User's Guide, Squires, Bricker, and Twombly. © 2002 Paul H. Brookes Publishing Co.

Figure B6.   If mail-out procedures are being used, staff can use the mail-out and mail-back master form provided with the ASQ:SE. The example shown here is ready to be mailed to Halle Moss's family for questionnaire completion.

Return Rates

As stated in Chapter 4, a common concern in using the questionnaires in the mail-out format is their return rate. Many screening programs use the questionnaires in this format, and a variety of ideas for increasing return rates have been generated. First, it is important to follow the steps for using the tracking system described previously. This includes making a follow-up telephone call a few days after the questionnaire is mailed to ensure receipt and to address any questions the parent might have. Many programs have found that this initial telephone call significantly increases return rates. If a questionnaire is not returned within 2 weeks, a second telephone call should be made to remind the parent to return the questionnaire. It is equally important to adhere to the tracking schedule for sending questionnaires and feedback. Parents should be able to expect the appropriate questionnaire on time and, after returning the questionnaire, should receive feedback in writing, by telephone, or in person within a short period. It may be important to include a welcome letter to parents with the first questionnaire, reminding them about the screening program and questionnaires.

A second option for increasing return rates is to provide incentives for parents. Incentives may be mailed to parents along with the feedback letter. For example, programs may find a local fast-food restaurant to sponsor the screening program by supplying coupons. Another idea is to include a birthday card with the questionnaires on the child's first, second, third, fourth, and fifth birthdays.

Third, staff may decide to mail a social-emotional activities guide, such as one of those provided in Appendix C of this *User's Guide,* with the feedback letter. These guides are designed to accompany each questionnaire and contain activities that parents may try at home.

Fourth, if resources permit, returning the questionnaires to the parents after staff have recorded scores may increase return rates by helping parents feel some "ownership" of the system.

When monitoring groups of children, a system must be created to alert program staff as to when activities (e.g., filling out a questionnaire, calling families to have questionnaires returned) should occur. A simple and inexpensive way is to create a card file tickler box, discussed previously in this appendix, although many programs may choose to develop their own system or utilize computer-based systems. In this appendix, the term *tickler system* refers to whatever system programs develop to help monitor screening activities.

Specific steps designed for the use and tracking of the mail-out ASQ:SE option are delineated next. Careful adherence to these steps is the first guideline for ensuring a high return rate.

1. Daily or once a week, a designated staff person should check the tickler system (i.e., card file or computer system), which indicates which children need a questionnaire completed in the next 1–2 weeks.

2. A staff member should copy the appropriate ASQ:SE age interval or remove a copy from the storage file, complete the identifying information on the first page of the questionnaire (including a contact person and telephone number for questions that may arise), and fill in the name of the administering program or provider on the second page of the questionnaire.

3. A target date for questionnaire completion (i.e., the date the child will be 6 months, 12 months, and so forth) should be entered into the tickler system.

4. The questionnaire should be prepared for mailing by stapling, by taping the ends, or by putting it in an envelope. If stapled or taped, the program's return address and a stamp should be added to the mail-out and mail-back sheet. If mailed in an envelope, a program-addressed, stamped envelope should be included.

5. Record the date the questionnaire is mailed in the tickler system.

6. Record in the tickler system a date to call the parent 3 or 4 days after mailing.

7. Check the tickler system and call parents on the date designated to ensure that the questionnaire was received and to answer any questions the parents may have about completing the questionnaire.

8. Record the date the parents were contacted in the tickler system.

9. If the questionnaire is returned before the expected return date, record the date returned in the tickler system.

10. If the questionnaire is not returned by the expected return date, call the child's parents and record the date in the tickler system.

11. Once a questionnaire is received, use the ASQ:SE Information Summary to score and compare scores with cutoffs.

12. If the questionnaire results indicate the child's social-emotional development appears to be typical, send a feedback letter like the one in Figure B7 (or for Spanish-speaking families, a letter like the one provided with the Spanish ASQ:SE questionnaires) and a social-emotional activities guide from Appendix C. If program resources permit, also send parents a copy of the completed questionnaire.

13. If the questionnaire results indicate that the child is identified as needing an in-depth assessment, call or arrange to meet with the child's parents to discuss the referral considerations outlined in the ASQ:SE Information Summary and to discuss options for follow-up.

    a. Ask the parents if they want the questionnaire results sent to their child's physician.

    b. When appropriate, obtain the parents' written consent to share questionnaire results with other agencies and the child's physician.

    c. Refer the child for further assessment, if indicated.

    d. Determine whether the child will continue to be monitored using the ASQ:SE questionnaires. Monitoring should be discontinued for three reasons: 1) at a parent's request, 2) if the child is older than 5 years, or 3) if social-emotional delays are identified

---

Dear [fill in parents' or guardians' names]:

Thank you for completing the *Ages & Stages Questionnaires: Social-Emotional* for your child. Your responses on the questionnaire show that your child's development appears to be progressing well.

Another questionnaire will be mailed to you in [fill in number here] months. Please remember again the importance of completing all items and of mailing the questionnaire back as soon as possible. Feel free to call if you have any questions. Thank you for your interest in our program.

Sincerely,

[fill in staff member's name]
[fill in program name]

The ASQ:SE User's Guide, Squires, Bricker, and Twombly. © 2002 Paul H. Brookes Publishing Co.

Figure B7.   A sample feedback letter to parents or guardians whose children's ASQ:SE scores indicate typical development. A Spanish translation of this letter is contained in Appendix G.

on the follow-up evaluation and the child begins receiving early intervention or mental health services.

14. If the child will continue to be monitored, enter the target date in tickler system to alert staff 1–2 weeks prior to the next questionnaire age interval.

INTERVIEWING PROCEDURES

A few things should be considered when interviewing families using the ASQ:SE. These steps are recommended for completing the ASQ:SE during an interview:

1. If necessary, obtain consent from the parent(s) for the child to participate in the monitoring program.

2. A copy of the age-appropriate questionnaire should be given or mailed to the parents prior to the interview so they can become familiar with the items and have a copy while being interviewed. Do not include the ASQ:SE Information Summary with the questionnaire.

3. Ask the parents for the identifying information on the second page of the questionnaire. The interviewer's name should be recorded along with the parents' names in the blank beside "Assisting in questionnaire completion."

4. Explain the purpose of the screening program, scoring options (*most of the time, sometimes, rarely or never*), and so forth that are outlined in the part of Chapter 4 called "Introducing the Screening Program to Parents."

5. Clarify the role of the interviewer (i.e., to read the items). Try not to influence parents' responses to items. Let them know you are interested in *their* feelings, observations, and opinions about their child's behavior.

6. Read each item on the questionnaire. While moving through the questionnaire items, the interviewer should identify the number of the question.

7. The interviewer should encourage maximum parental independence in completing the questionnaires, providing assistance only when necessary and using the time for communication about the child's social-emotional development.

8. If the parents are unsure of how to answer a question, offer to contact them later so that they have time to observe the child and think about the response.

9. The interviewer should remember that parents' comments are important and should be recorded.

10. Score the questionnaire with the parents using the ASQ:SE Information Summary. Respond as indicated in the section on ASQ:SE Referral Criteria in Chapter 4 of the *User's Guide.*

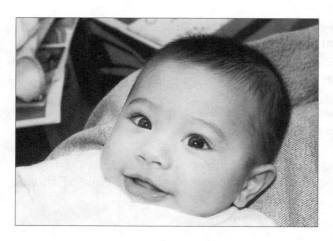

HOME VISITING PROCEDURES

The ASQ:SE can be adapted for use on home visits. As stated previously, it is important for the parents to understand the role of the home visitor: to help parents complete the questionnaires while being as nondirective as possible and offering support and assistance to clarify questions.

As mentioned previously, the ASQ:SE Information Summary, provided on the last page of each questionnaire, can be used on the home visit. This form can be completed by the home visitor to score the questionnaire, discuss referral considerations with parents, and provide immediate feedback and follow-up, if necessary.

The following list details the steps and decisions involved in implementing the ASQ:SE system while on a home visit:

1. If necessary, obtain consent from the parent(s) for the child to participate in the monitoring program.

2. Telephone and schedule a home visit date and time. Get directions to the family's home. Photocopy or remove from the file the language-appropriate (English or Spanish) and age-appropriate questionnaire. Questionnaires can be completed up to 3 months before or after the target age for the 6, 12, and 18 month ASQ:SE and up to 6 months before or after the target age for the 24, 36, 48, and 60 month ASQ:SE. Arrange for an interpreter if necessary.

3. Mail the language- and age-appropriate questionnaire to the child's home 1–2 weeks before the visit. In addition, bring a copy of the next questionnaire on the home visit, in case it is appropriate to leave it with the parent at the end of the visit (see Step 13 in this list).

4. Determine whether the parents are capable of reading and comprehending the questionnaire.
    a. *For parents who are unable to read or are otherwise unable to complete the questionnaire* (e.g., as a result of a developmental disability or a language difference)
        *   The home visitor may read the items on the questionnaire.
        *   The home visitor may describe the behaviors targeted by the question.
    b. *For parents who are able to read and comprehend the questionnaire*
        *   Parents can read and complete the questionnaire with the home visitor's assistance.

- The home visitor may help clarify what is meant by certain questions but should not assist parents in interpreting items.

5. To describe the questionnaire, the home visitor can give the following information:
   a. Description of the ASQ:SE system as a tool that parents and the home visitor can use to check the child's social-emotional development
   b. Clarification of the home visitor's role (i.e., to read and assist with understanding questions)

6. Begin the questionnaire by completing the second page (i.e., demographic information). If the home visitor is translating or assisting in the completion of the questionnaire (e.g., reading the questionnaire) or if an interpreter is present, this should be noted.

7. Explain the scoring system.
   a. *Most of the time* indicates the child is doing the behavior most of the time/too often.
   b. *Sometimes* indicates the child is doing the behavior occasionally but not consistently.
   c. *Rarely or never* indicates the child is not or is rarely doing the behavior.
   d. In addition, the parent may check items that are of concern to him or her.

8. Administer the questionnaire.
   a. If necessary, read each item.
   b. Encourage maximum parental independence in completing the questionnaires, providing assistance only when necessary.
   c. Paraphrase items as needed if parents need clarification.
   d. Highlight the child's strengths and reinforce positive parent–child interactions.
   e. If questions about cultural appropriateness of items come up during administration, discuss with the family (e.g., some cultures do not encourage eye contact).
   f. Try not to influence parents' responses to items. Let them know you are interested in their feelings, observations, and opinions about their child's behavior.
   g. If parents are unsure about a question, the home visitor can call parents in 1–2 weeks, thereby giving them more time to observe behaviors.

9. Complete the last few questions about eating/sleeping, general concerns, and things that the parents enjoy about the child, paying close attention to the parents' concerns.
   a. Offer suggestions and resources when appropriate.
   b. Encourage dialogue about the child's development and parenting issues.
   c. If interviewing a parent, record his or her comments carefully.

10. Score the questionnaire using the ASQ:SE Information Summary.
    a. The home visitor can do the scoring.
    b. Compare the child's score with the cutoff scores indicated on the ASQ:SE Information Summary.
11. Discuss the results with the parents.
    a. Encourage dialogue with the parents about the child's social-emotional development and any behaviors of concern.
    b. Discuss referral considerations (see ASQ:SE Information Summary) and possible follow-up options, when necessary.
12. Offer the list of age-appropriate social-emotional activities to families that is found in Appendix C.
    a. Describe some of the activities for the parents.
    b. Encourage the parents to place the list of activities in an accessible place (e.g., on the refrigerator door).
13. If appropriate, leave the next ASQ:SE interval as a guide for parents in observing their child's growth and development during the next 6–12 months.
14. Make arrangements for follow-up, referral, or the next home visit.

C

Social-Emotional Development and Activities Guide

ASQ:SE

The following social-emotional behavior development lists (on pp. 112–120) and activities (on pp. 121–129) coordinate with the ASQ:SE questionnaire intervals at 6, 12, 18, 24, 30, 36, 48 and 60 months. In addition, a social-emotional behavior development list and activities are included for birth to 6 months of age. After a child has been screened with the ASQ:SE and program staff have determined that there is no need to refer this child, staff may give the development lists and activities to the family as additional resources. The development lists are intended to provide parents with guidance about what types of behaviors they may expect from their growing child, while the activities provide ideas or ways to assist their young child's social-emotional development. Please consider the following points when using these resources.

First, the ASQ:SE development lists and activities

- May include behaviors or suggestions that are inappropriate for certain cultures
- *Are not an intervention.* Rather, these resources can be used in a preventive manner when children do not need further assessment.
- Should not be considered comprehensive
- May need to be modified to be appropriate for families (e.g., translated, shared verbally with families, illustrated)

Second, the following information, which is not included in the development lists or activities, should be made available to families. Parents may need support and/or information about developmentally appropriate expectations and strategies related to these topics to feel successful with their young children.

- Feeding young children (including breast feeding)
- Sleeping patterns
- Toilet training
- Guidance and discipline
- Safety and childproofing home environments
- Health and nutrition

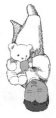

SOCIAL-EMOTIONAL BEHAVIOR DEVELOPMENT IN YOUNG CHILDREN

From birth to 6 months . . .

- When she is a newborn, your baby lets you know when she is hungry and uncomfortable by crying.

- Your baby often responds to your attempts to soothe him.

- Your baby likes to look at your face and will look in your eyes, but only for a couple of seconds at first.

- Your baby lets you know she is content by cooing.

- When he is a couple of months old, your baby lets you know he is happy by smiling, laughing, and gurgling.

- Your baby likes to be picked up, hugged, and cuddled by people she knows.

- Your baby enjoys being with other children and people and will sometimes be fussy just because he wants your attention.

- Around 5 months your baby will sometimes stop crying when you talk to her (rather than pick her up).

- Your baby likes to play with his fingers, hands, feet, and toes.

- She often holds onto you and enjoys your hugs.

- He recognizes familiar people by their voices.

- Your baby sometimes sucks on her fingers or hands to calm herself down.

The ASQ:SE User's Guide, Squires, Bricker, and Twombly. © 2002 Paul H. Brookes Publishing Co.

SOCIAL-EMOTIONAL BEHAVIOR DEVELOPMENT IN YOUNG CHILDREN

At 6 months . . .

- Your baby responds to your smile and is beginning to laugh when looking at you.

- Your baby is babbling or talking by putting sounds together such as "ma-ma-ma," "ba-ba-ba," and "da-da-da."

- Your baby responds to your soothing and comforting and loves to be touched or held close.

- Your baby responds to your affection and may begin to initiate signs of affection.

- Your baby enjoys watching other babies and children.

- Your baby tries to talk with noises and gurgles.

- Your baby focuses on your voice and turns her head to your voice. She may turn to you when you call her name.

- Your baby may be frightened by loud or unfamiliar noises.

- Your baby wants quiet and soothing sometimes and talking and playing at other times.

- Your baby enjoys simple games like Peekaboo or This Little Piggy.

- A lot of the time, your baby wants you and no one else!

The ASQ:SE User's Guide, Squires, Bricker, and Twombly. © 2002 Paul H. Brookes Publishing Co.

SOCIAL-EMOTIONAL BEHAVIOR DEVELOPMENT IN YOUNG CHILDREN

At 12 months (1 year) . . .

- Your baby responds to her name when you call her.

- Your baby is interested in other babies and children.

- Your baby is showing many emotions, such as happiness, sadness, discomfort, and anger.

- Your baby may be shy around new people and seem jealous if you pay attention to someone else. He may need some time to watch and warm up to new people and new places.

- Your baby may have fears such as of falling, darkness, large animals, loud sounds, or changes in routines.

- Your baby responds differently to strangers than she does to family members and friends that she sees a lot.

- Your baby wants you in his sight all of the time and may get upset when you leave him with someone else.

- Your baby is imitating other children and adults. She may imitate things such as sounds, actions, and facial expressions.

- Your baby gives affection by hugging and kissing people, pets, or stuffed animals.

- Your baby watches other people and may respond to someone's distress by crying or showing distress himself.

- Your baby is beginning to show her likes and dislikes and may push things away that she does not like. She may be attached to a special toy or blanket.

- Your baby is becoming more independent and may seem stubborn or frustrated when he can't do something himself.

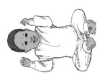

SOCIAL-EMOTIONAL BEHAVIOR DEVELOPMENT IN YOUNG CHILDREN

At 18 months . . .

- Your toddler is generally happy and smiles at people, including other children.
- Your toddler likes to talk and is using more words every day.
- Your toddler likes to show affection and give hugs and kisses.
- Your toddler may be showing different emotions such as fear, sympathy, modesty, guilt, or embarrassment.
- Your toddler likes to do things by himself. He may seem stubborn, but this is normal.
- Your toddler likes to help out with simple household tasks.
- Your toddler turns to you for help when she is in trouble.
- He enjoys playing near other children, but not with them yet.
- She may hand objects to other children, but she doesn't understand how to share and wants the toys right back.
- Your toddler can play by himself for short periods of time.
- Your toddler has specific likes and dislikes.
- Your toddler likes to say "No!" She may have a quick temper and sometimes hits when frustrated.
- Your toddler loves to be held and read to and becomes upset when separated from you.
- Your toddler loves to imitate others.
- Your toddler likes to be the center of attention.
- Your toddler recognizes himself in mirror or pictures.

The ASQ:SE User's Guide, Squires, Bricker, and Twombly. © 2002 Paul H. Brookes Publishing Co.

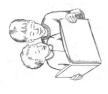

SOCIAL-EMOTIONAL BEHAVIOR DEVELOPMENT IN YOUNG CHILDREN

At 24 months (2 years) . . .

- Your toddler likes to imitate you, other adults, and her friends.

- Your toddler wants to do everything by himself, even though he can't!

- Your toddler's favorite words are "mine," "no," "me do it."

- Your toddler has a lot of emotions, and her emotions can be very "big." She can get angry and have temper tantrums.

- Your toddler likes to imitate household tasks and can put some of his toys away with help from you.

- Your toddler loves to try new things and explore new places but wants to know you are nearby to keep her safe.

- Your toddler is very interested in other children and is still learning how to play with them.

- He will play nearby other children, but not really with them. He doesn't understand how to share his things yet.

- Your toddler has a hard time waiting and wants things right now.

- Your toddler loves attention from familiar adults and children but may act shy around strangers.

- Your toddler is learning how to show affection by returning a hug or kiss. She tries to comfort familiar people who are in distress.

- Your toddler knows his name and knows what he likes and dislikes. He may be very attached to certain things such as a special book, toy, or blanket.

- Your toddler enjoys simple pretend play like pretending to cook or talk on the telephone.

- Your toddler is learning about the routines in your home, but generally she is unable to remember rules.

The ASQ:SE User's Guide, Squires, Bricker, and Twombly. © 2002 Paul H. Brookes Publishing Co.

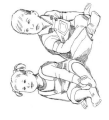

SOCIAL-EMOTIONAL BEHAVIOR DEVELOPMENT IN YOUNG CHILDREN

At 30 months . . .

- Your child enjoys playing alongside other children.

- He likes using his increasing imagination. Puppets, dress-up clothes, dolls, and play figures are fun playthings.

- Your child is beginning to understand others' feelings. She may be able to identify when another child is angry or happy.

- Your child is beginning to learn about sharing. He doesn't always share but can sometimes.

- Your child is getting louder and bossier at times. She may talk with a loud, urgent voice.

- Your child at this age can follow simple routine directions, such as "Bring me your cup" and "Please go in your room and get your socks."

- He enjoys hearing songs and stories—sometimes over and over again.

- Your child wants to be independent sometimes but also may want you nearby. She will now easily leave your side if she is in familiar surroundings.

- He can identify whether he is a boy or a girl.

- Your child may greet familiar adults and is happy to see familiar friends.

- She may scream and throw temper tantrums at times.

- He likes to be hugged and cuddled—but not in the middle of playtime.

The ASQ:SE User's Guide, Squires, Bricker, and Twombly. © 2002 Paul H. Brookes Publishing Co.

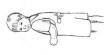

SOCIAL-EMOTIONAL BEHAVIOR DEVELOPMENT IN YOUNG CHILDREN

At 36 months (3 years) . . .

- There are many things your child can do for herself, and she will tell you, "I can do it myself!"

- Although he is more independent, your child is still learning to follow simple rules—and he may need gentle reminders.

- She now plays briefly *with* other children. She is learning more about sharing and taking turns.

- He may have a special friend that he prefers playing with. Boys may prefer playing with boys, and girls with girls.

- She is becoming more independent. When you go on outings, she won't always hold your hand and stay by your side.

- Your child's emotions may shift suddenly, from happy to sad, from mad to silly. He's trying to learn how to handle his emotions.

- She can sometimes express with words the feelings that she is having. She is beginning to think about the feelings of others and may be able to identify their feelings, too.

- Your child uses his imagination to create stories through pretend play with dolls, toy telephones, and action figures.

- Your child may boss people around and make demands. This shows not only that she is independent but also that she values herself. She might do something that is asked of her but may be more willing if she thinks it's her idea.

- Your child may be fearful and have nightmares. Television shows (even scary cartoons) can give him nightmares.

- Your child's attention span is increasing, and she often stays with an activity for at least 5 minutes.

The ASQ:SE User's Guide, Squires, Bricker, and Twombly. © 2002 Paul H. Brookes Publishing Co.

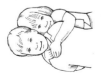

SOCIAL-EMOTIONAL BEHAVIOR DEVELOPMENT IN YOUNG CHILDREN

At 48 months (4 years) . . .

- Your child likes to play with other children and has favorite games and playmates.

- Your child is beginning to share and take turns but is possessive of favorite toys and playthings.

- Your child expresses extreme emotions at times—laughs, cries, is silly, angry. She may be able to label her own feelings.

- When your child plays, he often uses real-life situations such as going to the store, school, and gas station.

- Your child may continue to have imaginary friends when playing games, sleeping at night, and going to preschool.

- Your child now understands home rules if they are short and simple.

- Your child is starting to understand danger and knows when to stay away from dangerous things.

- Your child loves silly jokes and has a sense of humor.

- Your child is beginning to control her feelings of frustration.

- Your child may use his imagination a lot, and he can be very creative.

- Your child is becoming more independent and adventurous and may be attracted to try new things.

- With her new independence, your child may be boastful and bossy at times.

- Your child may show concern and sympathy for younger siblings and playmates when they're hurt or upset. His ability to empathize—to put himself in someone else's shoes—is increasing.

The ASQ:SE User's Guide, Squires, Bricker, and Twombly. © 2002 Paul H. Brookes Publishing Co.

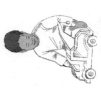

SOCIAL-EMOTIONAL BEHAVIOR DEVELOPMENT IN YOUNG CHILDREN

At 60 months (5 years) . . .

- Your child likes to play best with one or two other children at a time.

- He likes to choose his own friends and may have a best friend.

- Your child now plays simple table games like Candy Land and Lotto.

- Your child likes to play in small groups at the park or at school and may play with most of the children in her class.

- He understands and can follow simple rules at home and at school.

- Your child is showing a variety of emotions. She may be jealous of other children at times, especially of a younger brother or sister who is getting attention.

- Your child is now very independent and likes to make his own choices about clothes, foods to eat, and activities.

- Your child is sensitive to other children's feelings and can identify feelings in others: "He's sad."

- Your child likes to talk with familiar adults and children.

- Your child understands how to take turns and share at home and at school, but she may not want to all of the time.

- Your child is beginning to understand the meaning of right and wrong. He doesn't always do what is right, though.

- Adult approval is very important to your child. Your child looks to adults for recognition and acknowledgment.

- Your child is showing some self-control in group situations and can wait for her turn or stand in a line.

- Your child is usually able to respond to requests such as "Use your quiet voice" or "Inside is for walking."

- Your child's attention span is increasing. He is able to focus his attention for a necessary length of time such as when directions are being given or when a story is being read.

The ASQ:SE User's Guide, Squires, Bricker, and Twombly. © 2002 Paul H. Brookes Publishing Co.

SOCIAL-EMOTIONAL ACTIVITIES FOR INFANTS FROM BIRTH TO 6 MONTHS OLD

Sing lullabies and tell your baby nursery rhymes. Use a soft and gentle voice when you talk to him.	When your baby is a newborn, show her black-and-white pictures. Place them close to your baby (8–10 inches) so that she can look at them.	Let your baby hear new, gentle sounds. Quiet musical toys or soft bells will be interesting to him.	Hold your baby and look in her eyes and smile. Gently rub and touch her and tell her how much you love her.
If your baby cries, pick her up and tell her you love her. She may be hungry or uncomfortable.	Talk to your baby about things he is seeing, hearing, and feeling. Talk softly and gently to him during routines of the day.	Talk to your baby about things she seems to like or dislike. "You don't like that big noise, do you?"	Let your baby lie on a blanket on the floor and get down on the floor with him. See the world from his point of view.
Make life interesting for your baby. Introduce new sounds and places to him from the safety of your arms.	Praise your baby often. Tell her how strong she is getting and what a sweet girl she is. Tell her you love her.	Begin to play simple games with your baby such as Peekaboo. You can put a cloth over your head and peek out.	Introduce new, safe* objects for your baby to explore. Simple objects such as plastic cups and big wooden spoons are all new to her.
Place interesting objects on the wall close to your baby's bed or close to her line of vision. Simple pictures from magazines are great.	It's never too early to start reading books with your baby. Choose simple books first and talk about the pictures he sees. Cuddle up close.	Learn your baby's special language. She will "talk" to you with sounds and gestures and let you know when she is happy, uncomfortable, or hungry.	Gently rock your baby and dance with him to music. Your baby will love to move like this and be close to you.

*Be sure to review safety guidelines with your health care provider at each new age level.

The ASQ:SE User's Guide, Squires, Bricker, and Twombly. © 2002 Paul H. Brookes Publishing Co.

SOCIAL-EMOTIONAL ACTIVITIES FOR INFANTS 6 MONTHS OLD

Learn your baby's special routines, and try to settle into a consistent routine for eating, sleeping, and diapering. Talk to your baby about his routines. This will help your baby feel secure and content.	Your baby likes to hear new sounds. Bells, whistles, and barking dogs are all new and interesting. Talk to your baby about what she is hearing.	Get down on the floor with your baby and play with him on his level. Look at toys, books, or objects together. Have fun, laugh, and enjoy your special time together.	When your baby cries, respond to her. Whisper in her ear to quiet her. Hold her close and make soft sounds. This will help her know you are always there and that you love her.
Play Peekaboo and Pat-a-Cake with your baby. Be playful, have fun, and laugh with your baby. She will respond with smiles and laughs.	Read to your baby. Snuggle up close, point to pictures, and talk about what you are seeing. Your baby will begin to choose favorite books as he gets a bit older.	Bring your baby to new places to see new things. Go on a walk to a park or in the mall, or just bring her shopping. She will love to see new things while you keep her safe.	When you are working in your home, place your baby in new areas or in new positions. The world looks very different from a new spot!
Let your baby begin to feed himself bits of food and help feed himself with a spoon and a cup. He will begin to enjoy doing things by himself.	Use your baby's name when you dress, feed, and diaper her: "Here is Dusty's finger," "Here is Jen's foot."	Provide new objects for your baby to explore.* Everything is interesting to him. Plastic cups, large wooden spoons, and wet washcloths are all new and interesting.	"Talk" with your baby. When your baby makes a sound, imitate the sound back to her. Go back and forth as long as possible.
Sing songs to your baby and tell her nursery rhymes. Make up songs about your baby using her name. This will make her feel special and loved.	Bath time* is a wonderful time to have fun and be close with your baby. Sponges, plastic cups, and washcloths make simple, inexpensive tub toys.	Enjoy music with your baby. Pick her up, bounce gently, and twirl with her in your arms. Try new and different types of music to dance to.	Go over and visit a friend who has a baby or young child. Stay close to your baby and let him know that these new people are okay. It takes a little time to warm up.

*Be sure to review safety guidelines with your health care provider at each new age level.

The ASQ:SE User's Guide, Squires, Bricker, and Twombly. © 2002 Paul H. Brookes Publishing Co.

SOCIAL-EMOTIONAL ACTIVITIES FOR INFANTS 12 MONTHS OLD (1 YEAR OLD)

Keep a routine at home for eating, sleeping, diapering, and playtimes. Talk to your baby about routines and what will be next. This will help her feel secure.	Let your baby know how much you love him and how special he is every day—when he wakes up in the morning and when he goes to sleep at night.	Play simple games with your baby such as Pat-a-Cake, Peekaboo, and Hide and Seek, or chase each other. Laugh and have fun together!
While you are making dinner, your baby can "help." Have a drawer or cupboard that he can empty that is full of safe kitchen things such as measuring cups and big spoons.	Play gentle tickle games with your baby, but make sure to stop when she lets you know she has had enough. Watch her carefully and you will know.	Play name games with your baby like, "Where is Rita?"
Go on a walk to a park or a place where children play. Let your baby watch them and visit a little if she is ready.	Play with child-safe mirrors* with your baby. Make silly expressions and talk to your baby about what he is seeing in the reflection.	Dance to music with your baby. Hold his hands while he bends up and down. Clap and praise him when he "dances" by himself.
	Twirl your baby around. She will enjoy a little rough-and-tumble play, but make sure you stop when she has had enough.	Read together with your baby. Before naptime and bedtime is a great time to read together. Let your baby choose the book and snuggle up!
Let your baby have as many choices about foods, clothing, toys, and events as possible. He will enjoy making choices.	Sit on the floor with your baby and roll a ball back and forth. Clap your hands when your baby pushes the ball or "catches" the ball with his hands.	When you are dressing or diapering your baby, talk about her body parts and show her your body parts: "Here is Mommy's nose; here is Mary's nose."
Invite a friend over who has a baby or young child. Make sure you have enough toys for both children. It's a little early for them to know about sharing.		

*Be sure to review safety guidelines with your health care provider at each new age level.

The ASQ:SE User's Guide, Squires, Bricker, and Twombly. © 2002 Paul H. Brookes Publishing Co.

SOCIAL-EMOTIONAL ACTIVITIES FOR INFANTS 18 MONTHS OLD

Your toddler likes to have a consistent daily routine. Talk to him about what you are doing now and what will be happening next. Give him time to be active and time to be quiet.	Your toddler will enjoy gentle rough-housing and tickling games. Make sure he can let you know when he has had enough. He will like quiet snuggle-up times, too.	Have a pretend party with stuffed animals or dolls. You can cut out little "presents" from a magazine, make a pretend "cake," and sing the birthday song.
Your toddler needs a lot of time to move around and exercise.* Go for a walk to the park, visit a playground, or make a trip to a shopping mall.	Play simple games such as Hide and Seek and Chase with your toddler. Have fun and laugh together.	Dance with your toddler. Make a simple instrument out of a large plastic food tub (for a drum) or a small plastic container filled with beans or rice (for a shaker).
Your toddler will love to help out with daily tasks. Give him simple "jobs" to do and let him know what a big boy he is. He can wipe off a table, put his toys away, or help sweep up.	Let your toddler help out during meal-times by bringing some things to the table or setting a place.	Your child can help clean up after play-times. Make it simple by putting things in a big tub or box and help him clean. Clap and praise him for his help.
Help your child learn about emotions. In front of a mirror make happy faces, sad faces, mad faces, and silly faces. This is fun!	Your child might enjoy having a little place to hide. Use a blanket or sheet to make a tent or secret spot for her to play in.	Story times, especially before naptime and bedtime, are a great way to settle down before sleep. Let your child choose books to read and help her turn pages, and help her name what she sees.
Make playhouse furniture for your child out of boxes. For a stove, turn a box upside down and draw "burners." Some plastic containers make safe pots, and wooden spoons stir the soup.	Set up playtimes with other children. Your child doesn't understand how to share yet, so make sure there are plenty of toys. Stay close by and help her learn how to play with other children.	Your toddler is getting big and wants to do things by himself! Let him practice eating with a spoon and drinking with a tippy cup during mealtimes. Get ready for some spilling!

*Be sure to review safety guidelines with your health care provider at each new age level.

The ASQ:SE User's Guide, Squires, Bricker, and Twombly. © 2002 Paul H. Brookes Publishing Co.

SOCIAL-EMOTIONAL ACTIVITIES FOR INFANTS 24 MONTHS OLD (2 YEARS OLD)

Try to have clear routines during the day, and let your child know what will be happening next. "Remember, after we brush hair, we get dressed."	Your child is learning about rules but will need lots and lots of reminders. Keep rules short and simple, and be consistent.	Have a special reading time every day with your toddler. Snuggle up and get close. Before bedtimes or naptimes is a great time to read together.	Let your toddler know how special she is! She will love to be praised for new things she learns how to do: "You are so helpful," "Wow, you did it yourself!"
When your child plays with friends, stay nearby to help them learn about taking turns. It is still early for your child to know how to share, but talking about turns will help her learn.	Give your toddler choices, but keep them simple. While dressing, let him choose a red or a blue shirt. At lunch, let him choose milk or juice.	Provide lots of time to play with other children. Your child will play hard but needs rest times too. Try to learn your child's rhythms and go with her flow.	Let your child do more things for himself.* Put a stool near the sink so he can wash his hands and brush his teeth. Let him pick out clothes and help dress himself.
Get down on the floor and play with your child. Try to follow your child's lead by playing with toys he wants to play with and trying his ideas.	Encourage your child to pretend play. With plastic cups, plastic containers, and some spoons, you can make some yummy "soup." Praise your toddler's cooking.	Everything is new to your toddler. She can find beauty in the little things like some weeds growing on a path or a pigeon pecking for seeds. Take some time to see the little things with her.	Your toddler is learning all about emotions. Help him label his feelings when he is mad, sad, happy, or silly: "You are really happy," "You seem really mad."
Play Parade or Follow the Leader with your toddler. Your child will love to copy you—and be the leader!	If your child has a temper tantrum, stay calm and talk in a quiet tone. If possible, ignore her until she calms down by herself.	Don't forget to tell your child how much you love him! Give him hugs and kisses and soft touches to let him know.	Teach your child simple songs like "Eensy Weensy Spider" where she can use her fingers.

*Be sure to review safety guidelines with your health care provider at each new age level.

The ASQ:SE User's Guide, Squires, Bricker, and Twombly. © 2002 Paul H. Brookes Publishing Co.

SOCIAL-EMOTIONAL ACTIVITIES FOR YOUNG CHILDREN 30 MONTHS OLD

Make a "Me Book" with your child. Take some pieces of paper and glue in pictures of your child, family members, pets, or other special things. Tape the pages together.	Tell your child funny stories about things he did when he was a baby. Begin a favorite story and see if he can tell what happens next.	Show your child family photos. Talk about the people in the pictures and who they are: "That's your Uncle Joe." Can your child tell you who the people are?	Tell your child a favorite nursery rhyme and ask her how the characters in the story felt.
Give your child directions that have two steps, like "Put all of the Legos in the box, and then put the box away in the closet." Let her know what a big help she is!	When cooking and cleaning, let your child help.* He can do things like helping to stir, putting flour in a cup, or putting away spoons and forks in the drawer.	Your child loves to imitate you. Try new words, animal sounds, and noises, and see if your child can imitate what you say or how you sound.	Encourage creative play, such as drawing with crayons, painting, and playing with playdough. Playing with chalk on the sidewalk is fun.
Let your child do more things for himself. Put a step stool near the bathroom sink so he can wash his hands and brush his teeth.	Draw and cut out different "feeling" faces, such as angry, frustrated, and happy. Encourage your child to use the faces to tell you how she is feeling.	Every day, tell your child how much you love him. Give him big hugs and little hugs, big kisses and little kisses.	Have a special reading time every day. Snuggle up and get close. Before bedtimes and naptimes is a great time to read together.
Play with your child and help her learn how to share. Show her how to share and praise her when she shares with you. This is a new thing for her, so don't expect too much at this age.	Encourage your child to tell you his name and age. Sometimes making up a rhyme or song about his name will help him remember. See if he can tell you the name of his friends and teachers.	Sing songs and dance with your child. Play different types of music from the radio. Make simple instruments from boxes, oatmeal cans, or yogurt tubs.	Take your child to a park and play with her near other children. She may just watch children at first but will join in with others when she is ready.

*Be sure to review safety guidelines with your health care provider at each new age level.

The ASQ:SE User's Guide, Squires, Bricker, and Twombly. © 2002 Paul H. Brookes Publishing Co.

SOCIAL-EMOTIONAL ACTIVITIES FOR YOUNG CHILDREN 36 MONTHS OLD (3 YEARS OLD)

Tell your child a simple story about something she did that was funny or interesting. See if your child can tell a different story about herself.	Encourage your child to identify and label his emotions and those of other children or adults.	Provide opportunities for your child to play with other children in your neighborhood or at a park.*	Many children this age have imaginary friends. Let your child talk and play with these pretend playmates.
Give your child choices. For example, when dressing, let him choose between two shirts or during snack time, let him choose between two snacks.	When you and your child are cooking, dressing, or cleaning,* give her directions that have at least two steps: "Put that pan in the sink and then pick up the red spoon."	Write a letter together to grandparents, a pen pal, or friend. See if your child can tell you what to write about himself to include in the letter.	Play games with your child that involve taking turns, such as Follow the Leader and Hopscotch.
With stuffed animals or dolls, create conflict situations. Talk with your child about what happened, feelings, and how best to work out problems when they come up.	Have a special reading time each day. Snuggle up and get close. Slowly increase the length of the stories so your child can sit and listen a little longer.	Every day, let your child know you love her and how great she is. Give her a "high five," a big smile, a pat on the back, or a hug. Tell her she is super, cool, sweet, and fun.	Tell your child a favorite story such as the Three Little Pigs or Goldilocks and the Three Bears. See if your child can tell you how the animals felt in the story.
Draw and cut out different feeling faces, and then glue them on Popsicle sticks. Let your child act out the different feelings with the puppets.	Get down on the floor and play with your child. Try to follow your child's lead by playing with toys he wants to play with and trying his ideas.	Play games such as Mother May I and Red Light, Green Light that involve following simple directions.	Tell silly jokes with your child. Simple "What am I?" riddles are also fun. Have a good time and laugh with your child.

*Be sure to review safety guidelines with your health care provider at each new age level.

The ASQ:SE User's Guide, Squires, Bricker, and Twombly. © 2002 Paul H. Brookes Publishing Co.

SOCIAL-EMOTIONAL ACTIVITIES FOR YOUNG CHILDREN 48 MONTHS OLD (4 YEARS OLD)

Introduce a new feeling each day using pictures, gestures, and words. Encourage your child to use a variety of words to describe how he feels.	Encourage activities that involve sharing, such as blocks, crayons, playdough, acting out stories. Give your child lots of time to play with other children.	Provide opportunities for your child to be creative. Empty containers, glue, newspapers, rubber bands, and magazines can be used for making new inventions.	Take your child to the store, to a restaurant or the library. Explore lots of new places.* Talk with her about similarities and differences in people.
When doing housework or yard work, allow your child to do a small part on her own. Let her empty the wastebasket or clean crumbs off the table.	Talk with your child about possible dangers in your home, such as electrical outlets and stovetops. Talk about outdoor dangers, too, such as crossing the street or talking with strangers.*	Encourage your child's independence. Let him fix a sandwich like peanut butter and jelly. At bedtime, let him choose his clothes to wear the next day.	Develop a conflict or argument with stuffed animals or puppets. Talk first about how the different animals are feeling. Discuss with your child how to resolve the conflict.
Tell a favorite nursery rhyme or story. Talk about what is make-believe and what is real.	Using stuffed animals or play figures, create a party or group playtime. Play different people and talk about how they might feel and act.	Tell a favorite nursery rhyme or story about "anger," and talk about positive ways the characters in the story resolved their differences.	Take your child to the library for story hour. She can learn about sitting in a group and listening to stories.
Your child is learning more about rules but will still need reminders. Talk about your family rules. Keep rules short and simple, and be consistent.	Have simple props like old clothes, boxes, and plastic utensils for playing store, fire station, and school.	Remember at least once a day to hug and cuddle and to praise your child for new skills—independence, creativity, expressing emotions, and sharing toys.	Try to have clear routines during the day, and let your child know what will happen next. Have a reading time and quiet time each day.

*Be sure to review safety guidelines with your health care provider at each new age level.

The ASQ:SE User's Guide, Squires, Bricker, and Twombly. © 2002 Paul H. Brookes Publishing Co.

SOCIAL-EMOTIONAL ACTIVITIES FOR YOUNG CHILDREN 60 MONTHS OLD (5 YEARS OLD)

Tell simple jokes and riddles. Your child will love it when you laugh at her jokes. The sillier, the better.	Gather old shirts, skirts, hats, and so forth from friends or a thrift store. Encourage dramatic play—acting out stories, songs, and scenes from the neighborhood.	Most of the time, your child will feel good about doing small jobs around the house.* Give her a lot of praise when she does a good job, and tell her what a big help she is.
Your child may need some help resolving conflicts, especially with his friends. Let him know he should use his words but can come to you for help.	Make sure your child has plenty of rest and quiet and alone time when she needs it.	Tell your child a favorite nursery rhyme that involves the idea of "right" and "wrong," and discuss what kinds of choices the characters made in the story.
Let your child know how special she is. Give her a lot of love, praise, and hugs every day.	Show your child pictures cut out from magazines of people from different cultures. Talk about things that are the same or different between your family and other families.	Play games with your child. Board games or card games that have three or more rules are great. Go Fish, Checkers, or Candy Land are examples.
Have a special time for reading each day. Snuggle up and get close. Before bedtime is a great time to read together.	Using hand-drawn pictures or pictures cut out from a magazine, talk about real dangers (fire, guns, cars) and make-believe dangers (monsters under the bed, the dark).	Build a store, house, puppet stage, or fire truck out of old boxes. Your child can invite a friend over to play store or house, have a puppet show, or be firefighters.
		Encourage your child to talk about the different rules at home and at school. Talk about why we have rules.

*Be sure to review safety guidelines with your health care provider at each new age level.

The ASQ:SE User's Guide, Squires, Bricker, and Twombly. © 2002 Paul H. Brookes Publishing Co.

D

Case Studies

ROBERT, 36 MONTHS OLD

Robert, who is 3 years old, lives most of the week with his younger sister and his 18-year-old mother, Margaret. Robert is an active young boy who is fascinated by big machines such as tractors and backhoes and likes to use toy machines to build roads. He loves to make his little sister laugh and is often quite silly. Robert's mother lives in a rural area, many miles from the nearest store or neighbor, and receives services from a home-visiting program for high school–age parents. Robert's father, Dell, lives 45 minutes away with his wife and her four children. Robert stays with his father 2 days a week, where he is taken care of by his paternal grandmother.

Gloria, the home visitor, brought the 36 month ASQ:SE to complete with Margaret through an interview. While her main purpose in visiting Margaret is to assist her in completing high school, the home visitor also monitors and screens the development of Robert and his sister. After Margaret completed the 36 month questionnaire, Gloria reviewed Margaret's answers and scored the questionnaire using the ASQ:SE Information Summary. Robert's score was high (105 points), well above the suggested 59-point cutoff for referral on the 36 month interval. After reviewing the questionnaire (see the completed questionnaire in Figure D1), Gloria spent some time talking with Margaret about the following referral considerations outlined on the ASQ:SE Information Summary.

Setting/Time Factors

Robert is not currently in preschool; he has two different home environments. From the questionnaire, it is clear from Question 31 that many people have expressed concerns about Robert's angry behaviors. Margaret wrote in the comments section that "everyone, grandparents, aunts, uncles" have expressed concerns. Gloria suggested to Margaret that Robert's father complete an ASQ:SE.

131

Left panel (page 3)

Please read each question carefully and
1. Check the box ☐ that best describes your child's behavior and
2. Check the circle ○ if this behavior is a concern

#	Question	MOST OF THE TIME	SOMETIMES	RARELY OR NEVER	CHECK IF THIS IS A CONCERN
1.	Does your child look at you when you talk to her?	☑ z 0	☐ v	☐ x	○
2.	Does your child like to be hugged or cuddled?	☑ z 0	☐ v	☐ x	○
3.	Does your child talk and/or play with adults he knows well?	☑ z 0	☐ v	☐ x	○
4.	Does your child cling to you more than you expect?	☐ x	☑ v 5	☐ z	○
5.	When upset, can your child calm down within 15 minutes?	☐ z	☐ v	☑ x 10	○
6.	Does your child seem too friendly with strangers?	☐ x	☑ v 5	☐ z	○
7.	Can your child settle herself down after periods of exciting activity?	☐ z	☑ v 5	☐ x	○
8.	Can your child move from one activity to the next with little difficulty, such as from playtime to mealtime?	☑ z 0	☐ v	☐ x	○
9.	Does your child seem happy?	☑ z 0	☐ v	☐ x	○

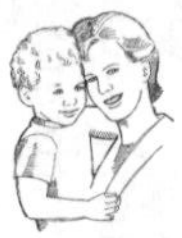

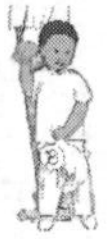

TOTAL POINTS ON PAGE __25__

Ages & Stages Questionnaires: Social-Emotional, Squires et al.
© 2002 Paul H. Brookes Publishing Co.   3

ASQ:SE   36 months/3 years

Right panel (page 4)

#	Question	MOST OF THE TIME	SOMETIMES	RARELY OR NEVER	CHECK IF THIS IS A CONCERN
10.	Is your child interested in things around him such as people, toys, and foods?	☑ z 0	☐ v	☐ x	○
11.	Does your child do what you ask her to do?	☐ z	☑ v 5	☐ x	○
12.	Does your child seem more active than other children her age?	☑ x 10	☐ v	☐ z	○
13.	Can your child stay with activities she enjoys for at least 5 minutes (not including watching television)?	☑ z 0	☐ v	☐ x	○
14.	Do you and your child enjoy mealtimes together?	☑ z 0	☐ v	☐ x	○
15.	Does your child have eating problems, such as stuffing foods, vomiting, eating nonfood items, or _____? (You may write in another problem.)	☐ x	☐ v	☑ z 0	○
16.	Does your child sleep at least 8 hours in a 24-hour period?	☑ z 0	☐ v	☐ x	○
17.	Does your child use words to tell you what he wants or needs?	☑ z 0	☐ v	☐ x	○

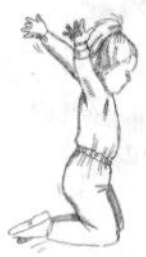

TOTAL POINTS ON PAGE __15__

Ages & Stages Questionnaires: Social-Emotional, Squires et al.
© 2002 Paul H. Brookes Publishing Co.   4

ASQ:SE   36 months/3 years

Figure D1.   36 month ASQ:SE for Robert. Robert's mother Margaret completed this ASQ:SE in an interview with a home visitor.

Questions 18–25

	MOST OF THE TIME	SOMETIMES	RARELY OR NEVER	CHECK IF THIS IS A CONCERN
18. Does your child follow routine directions? For example, does she come to the table or help clean up her toys when asked?	☐z	☐v	☑x 10	☑ 5
19. Does your child cry, scream, or have tantrums for long periods of time?	☐x	☑v 5	☐z	○
20. Does your child check to make sure you are near when exploring new places, such as a park or a friend's home?	☑z 0	☐v	☐x	○
21. Does your child do things over and over and can't seem to stop? Examples are rocking, hand flapping, spinning, or *yelling, fighting, doesn't listen to his mother* (You may write in something else.)	☐x	☑v 5	☐z	○
22. Does your child hurt himself on purpose?	☐x	☐v	☑z 0	○
23. Does your child stay away from dangerous things, such as fire and moving cars?	☐z	☐v	☑x 10	○
24. Does your child destroy or damage things on purpose?	☐x	☑v 5	☐z	○
25. Does your child use words to describe her feelings and the feelings of others, such as, "I'm happy," "I don't like that," or "She's sad"?	☑z 0	☐v	☐x	○

TOTAL POINTS ON PAGE 40

ASQ:SE 36 months/3 years

Ages & Stages Questionnaires: Social-Emotional, Squires et al.
© 2002 Paul H. Brookes Publishing Co.

5

Questions 26–32

	MOST OF THE TIME	SOMETIMES	RARELY OR NEVER	CHECK IF THIS IS A CONCERN
26. Can your child name a friend?	☑z 0	☐v	☐x	○
27. Do *other* children like to play with your child? *If they are not fighting*	☐z	☑v 5	☐x	○
28. Does *your child* like to play with other children?	☑z 0	☐v	☐x	○
29. Does your child try to hurt other children, adults, or animals (for example, by kicking or biting)?	☐x	☐v	☑z 0	○
30. Does your child show an interest in or knowledge of sexual language and activity?	☐x	☑v 5	☐z	○
31. Has anyone expressed concerns about your child's behaviors? If you checked "sometimes" or "most of the time," please explain: *Everybody—Grandparents, aunts, uncles*	☑x 10	☐v	☐z	☑ 5
32. Do you have any concerns about your child's eating, sleeping, or toileting habits? If so, please explain: *No*				○

TOTAL POINTS ON PAGE 25

ASQ:SE 36 months/3 years

Ages & Stages Questionnaires: Social-Emotional, Squires et al.
© 2002 Paul H. Brookes Publishing Co.

6

(continued)

Figure D1. (continued)

134

33. Is there anything that worries you about your child? If so, please explain:

His behavior

34. What things do you enjoy most about your child?

He loves his sister and plays with her.

---

36 Month/3 Year ASQ:SE Information Summary

Child's name: *Robert Mendez*
Person filling out the ASQ:SE: *Margaret Mendez*
Mailing address: *76 Blair Drive*
Telephone: *555-7751*
Today's date: *9-6-01*

Child's date of birth: *8-10-98*
Relationship to child: *Mother*
City: *Ocean Valley*   State: *CA*   zip:
Assisting in ASQ:SE completion: *Gloria*
Administering program/provider: *Oregon Valley EI*

SCORING GUIDELINES

1. Make sure the parent has answered all questions and has checked the concern column as necessary. If all questions have been answered, go to Step 2. If not all questions have been answered, you should first try to contact the parent to obtain answers or, if necessary, calculate an average score (see pages 39 and 41 of *The ASQ:SE User's Guide*).

2. Review any parent comments. If there are no comments, go to Step 3. If a parent has written in a response, see the section titled "Parent Comments" on pages 39, 41, and 42 of *The ASQ:SE User's Guide* to determine if the response indicates a behavior that may be of concern.

3. Using the following point system:

   Z (for zero) next to the checked box = 0 points
   V (for Roman numeral V) next to the checked box = 5 points
   X (for Roman numeral X) next to the checked box = 10 points
   Checked concern = 5 points

   Add together:

   Total points on page 3 = 25
   Total points on page 4 = 15
   Total points on page 5 = 40
   Total points on page 6 = 25

   Child's total score = 105

SCORE INTERPRETATION

1. *Review questionnaires*
   Review the parent's answers to questions. Give special consideration to any individual questions that score 10 or 15 points and any written or verbal comments that the parent shares. Offer guidance, support, and information to families, and refer if necessary, as indicated by score and referral considerations.

2. *Transfer child's total score*
   In the table below, enter the child's total score (transfer total score from above).

Questionnaire interval	Cutoff score	Child's ASQ:SE score
36 months/3 years	59	105

3. *Referral criteria*
   Compare the child's total score with the cutoff in the table above. If the child's score falls above the cutoff and the factors in Step 4 have been considered, refer the child for a mental health evaluation.

4. *Referral considerations*
   It is always important to look at assessment information in the context of other factors influencing a child's life. Consider the following variables prior to making referrals for a mental health evaluation. Refer to pages 44–46 in *The ASQ:SE User's Guide* for additional guidance related to these factors and for suggestions for follow-up.

   • Setting/time factors
     (e.g., Is the child's behavior the same at home as at school? Have there been any stressful events in the child's life recently?)

   • Development factors
     (e.g., Is the child's behavior related to a developmental stage or a developmental delay?)

   • Health factors
     (e.g., Is the child's behavior related to health or biological factors?)

   • Family/cultural factors
     (e.g., Is the child's behavior acceptable given cultural or family context?)

Developmental Factors

Gloria also had Margaret complete the 36 month ASQ. On this developmental screening tool, Robert's scores were well above the cutoffs, indicating typical development. Gloria felt that she could rule out a developmental delay as the cause of Robert's behavior. While Robert is an active 3-year-old boy, many of his behaviors identified on the ASQ:SE are not typical of 3-year-old children. For example, the ASQ:SE indicates that Robert is rarely able to calm himself within 15 minutes, rarely able to follow routine directions, and rarely stays away from dangerous things. These behaviors are not usually seen in 3-year-old children, and Robert's family is justly concerned about them.

Health Factors

In terms of overall health, Robert has not had a medical checkup for almost 6 months. Margaret was not certain if Robert had had his hearing or vision checked in the past. The family does not always follow a routine, and Robert's schedule changes depending on where he is staying for the night. Lack of sleep may be contributing to Robert's behaviors.

Family/Cultural Factors

Gloria did not believe that Robert's scores on the ASQ:SE were influenced by the family's culture. However, both Margaret and Gloria thought that Robert's behavior may be related to the stress he is under—having to travel between two homes and having two different sets of rules to understand. In addition, Margaret talked about feeling isolated and depressed. Although Margaret's mother helps her with rides and running errands, lack of transportation has been a real problem for Margaret. Gloria thought Robert's behavior might also be in part a reaction to not enough attention/responsiveness from his mother.

Follow-Up

Gloria discussed the results of the ASQ:SE with Margaret and talked to her about having Robert receive further evaluation. However, Margaret was not willing to take this step. Margaret applied to a child care program for low-income families that Robert will qualify for in 5 months. This program will provide transportation for Robert to and from the child care setting. Once Robert is in the child care program, Gloria plans on revisiting the topic of an evaluation with Margaret if Robert's behavior has not significantly improved. In this subsidized child care program, Robert will be able to receive a mental health evaluation and have access to services such as play therapy. Gloria decided that the best she could do until then was to follow up on some of the ASQ:SE referral considerations:

- Margaret did agree to have Robert have a health check-up and to discuss Robert's behaviors with his primary health care provider. Margaret agreed to set up an appointment, and Gloria agreed to help Margaret with finding transportation.

- Over the next few months, Gloria made plans to provide information and support to Margaret about a variety of topics related to behavior including the importance of Robert's eating a well-balanced diet, the importance of routines in a child's day, and how Robert needs to have enough sleep every night. Gloria will share activities with Margaret from the ASQ:SE that have been designed to promote healthy social-emotional behaviors in children Robert's age (see Appendix C). Gloria received some relevant information from a local early childhood specialist on positive parenting information that will be particularly helpful to Margaret in focusing on Robert's tantrums and learning about safety in the home.

- Margaret mentioned that she would like to go to church but hadn't been able to find a way to get there. Gloria encouraged Margaret to call the church, and Margaret was able to find transportation for herself and the children on Sundays. This action is a start to getting Margaret out in the community. Margaret is interested in learning how to drive and getting a car. Gloria wants to support and encourage Margaret to continue pursuing these goals.

- Gloria attempted to schedule a meeting with Robert's father, Dell, but he stated that "nothing is wrong" with Robert and that he didn't have time to meet with her. Dell did give Gloria permission to talk to Robert's grandmother, who takes care of Robert during the day when the boy stays at Dell's home. Margaret had talked to her, and she had said she was having a hard time with some of Robert's behaviors. Gloria hopes to share information with Robert's grandmother about positive behavior management strategies.

While Gloria feels that the plan that she and Margaret have built is a good beginning, she still feels that both Robert and Margaret would benefit from receiving services from a mental health or behavior specialist. Gloria would like to see Robert and Margaret go to counseling together, especially since much of Robert's anger and violent behavior is directed toward Margaret. She plans on revisiting the topic of evaluation and counseling with Margaret once Robert enters child care.

JOHN, 30 MONTHS OLD

John, 30 months old, lives with his mother, Juanita, and father, Manuel, three older siblings, his grandmother, and an aunt. John loves to be with his older siblings, who help take care of him. John enjoys singing songs with his mother and grandmother and reading books about animals. Manuel loves his son and wrestles and plays with John when he is home, although he works long hours. Four months ago Juanita took a job outside of the home. Juanita's mother took care of John and his older siblings during the day, but 2 months ago, Juanita's mother became ill, and Juanita scrambled to find child care. John was placed in a local child care setting and has had an extremely difficult time adjusting to this new setting. Both the child care provider and Juanita have expressed concerns about his behavior.

Lois is a family advocate who provides home visits to the family for a Part C early intervention provider. After hearing Juanita's concerns about John's behavior, Lois met Juanita at John's child care and brought the 30 month ASQ:SE to complete. Lois reviewed Juanita's answers and scored the questionnaire using the ASQ:SE Information Summary. John's score was 80 points, over the cutoff of 57. After reviewing the questionnaire (see the completed questionnaire in Figure D2), Lois encouraged Juanita and the child care provider to discuss the referral considerations outlined on the ASQ:SE Information Summary.

Setting/Time Factors

John's behavior appeared to be problematic mostly at school, although Juanita had seen some behavioral changes at home, especially during mealtimes. Juanita also stated that since John started going to child care, at home he almost never wants to be put down or for Juanita or another family member to be out of his sight. Juanita said she felt like she has a lot of added responsibilities and cannot always attend to John.

Developmental Factors

John was born 3 months premature and was carried by family members during most of his first year. He didn't begin walking until he was 2 years old. John recently became eligible for Part C early intervention services due to delays in his gross and fine motor skills, although he was found to have typical cognitive and adaptive skills. His communication skills were low but not low enough to make him eligible for speech-language services. The early intervention evaluator believed that John's delay in communication might be due to speaking both English and Spanish at home.

Health Factors

John had a checkup with his primary health care provider at 24 months and was found to be healthy, although Juanita has not discussed her concerns about mealtimes with the doctor. Juanita noted on the ASQ:SE that when John gets angry or upset while eating, he vomits. This behavior has been happening more frequently both at home and at school in the last 2 months.

Family/Cultural Factors

John is of Mexican descent. His mother and father are bilingual, and his grandmother only speaks Spanish. The child care provider speaks English and has had difficulty understanding John, who speaks a mixture of English and Spanish.

Please read each question carefully and
1. Check the box ☐ that best describes your child's behavior *and*
2. Check the circle ○ if this behavior is a concern

	MOST OF THE TIME	SOMETIMES	RARELY OR NEVER	CHECK IF THIS IS A CONCERN
1. Does your child look at you when you talk to him?	☑ z	☐ v	☐ x	○
2. Does your child like to be hugged or cuddled?	☑ z	☐ v	☐ x	○
3. Does your child cling to you more than you expect?	☑ x 10	☐ v	☐ z	○
4. Does your child greet or say hello to familiar adults?	☑ z	☐ v	☐ x	○
5. Does your child seem happy?	☑ z	☐ v	☐ x	○
6. Does your child like to hear stories and sing songs?	☑ z	☐ v	☐ x	○
7. Does your child seem too friendly with strangers?	☐ x	☐ v	☑ z	○
8. Does your child seem more active than other children her age?	☐ x	☐ v	☑ z	○
9. Can your child settle himself down after periods of exciting activity?	☐ z	☑ v 5	☐ x	○
10. Does your child cry, scream, or have tantrums for long periods of time?	☑ x 10	☐ v	☐ z	○
11. Does your child do things over and over and can't seem to stop? Examples are rocking, hand flapping, spinning, or _____ (You may write in something else.)	☐ x	☐ v	☑ z	○

TOTAL POINTS ON PAGE 25

ASQ:SE   30 months

	MOST OF THE TIME	SOMETIMES	RARELY OR NEVER	CHECK IF THIS IS A CONCERN
12. Can your child stay with activities she enjoys for at least 3 minutes (not including watching television)?	☑ z	☐ v	☐ x	○
13. Does your child do what you ask him to do?	☐ z	☑ v 5	☐ x	○
14. Is your child interested in things around her, such as people, toys, and foods?	☑ z	☐ v	☐ x	○
15. When upset, can your child calm down within 15 minutes?	☐ z	☑ v 5	☐ x	○
16. Does your child have eating problems such as stuffing foods, vomiting, eating nonfood items, or _when angry he vomits_ ? (You may write in another problem.)	☑ x 10	☐ v	☐ z	☑ 5
17. Do you and your child enjoy mealtimes together?	☑ z	☐ v	☐ x	○
18. When you point at something, does your child look in the direction you are pointing?	☑ z	☐ v	☐ x	○
19. Does your child sleep at least 8 hours in a 24-hour period?	☑ z	☐ v	☐ x	○
20. Does your child let you know how he is feeling with either words or gestures? For example, does he let you know when he is hungry, hurt, or tired?	☑ z	☐ v	☐ x	○

TOTAL POINTS ON PAGE 25

ASQ:SE   30 months

Figure D2. 30 month ASQ:SE for John. John's mother completed this ASQ:SE.

	MOST OF THE TIME	SOMETIMES	RARELY OR NEVER	CHECK IF THIS IS A CONCERN
21. Does your child follow routine directions? For example, does she come to the table or help clean up her toys when asked?	☑ z	☐ v	☐ x	○
22. Does your child check to make sure you are near when exploring new places, such as a park or a friend's home?	☑ z	☐ v	☐ x	○
23. Can your child move from one activity to the next with little difficulty, such as from playtime to mealtime? *at home he does, but not at child care*	☐ z	☑ v 5	☐ x	○
24. Does your child stay away from dangerous things, such as fire and moving cars?	☑ z	☐ v	☐ x	○
25. Does your child destroy or damage things on purpose?	☐ x	☑ v 5	☐ z	○
26. Does your child hurt himself on purpose?	☐ x	☐ v	☑ z	○
27. Does your child play alongside other children?	☐ z	☑ v 5	☐ x	○
28. Does your child try to hurt other children, adults, or animals (for example, by kicking or biting)?	☐ x	☐ v	☑ z	○

TOTAL POINTS ON PAGE 15

ASQ:SE 5   30 months

Ages & Stages Questionnaires: Social-Emotional; Squires et al.
© 2002 Paul H. Brookes Publishing Co.

	MOST OF THE TIME	SOMETIMES	RARELY OR NEVER	CHECK IF THIS IS A CONCERN
29. Has anyone expressed concerns about your child's behaviors? If you checked "sometimes" or "most of the time," please explain: *can't seem to adjust to childcare* *can't separate from me and family members*	☑ x 10	☐ v	☐ z	☑ 5
30. Do you have concerns about your child's eating and sleeping behaviors or about her toilet training? If so, please explain: *I worry about him choking on food sometimes.*				
31. Is there anything that worries you about your child? If so, please explain: *One thing that worries me is his difficulty adjusting to child care.*				
32. What things do you enjoy most about your child? *He's silly and laughs a lot.*				

TOTAL POINTS ON PAGE 15

ASQ:SE 6   30 months

(continued)

Ages & Stages Questionnaires: Social-Emotional; Squires et al.
© 2002 Paul H. Brookes Publishing Co.

Figure D2. *(continued)*

30 Month ASQ:SE Information Summary

Child's name: _John Jones_   Child's date of birth: _3-10-99_
Person filling out the ASQ:SE: _Juanita Jones_   Relationship to child: _Mother_
Mailing address: _7605 Park Street._   City: _Dexter_   State: _IL_   ZIP: _____
Telephone: _555-8665_   Assisting in ASQ:SE completion: _Lois_
Today's date: _9-18-01_   Administering program/provider: _Family Connections_

SCORING GUIDELINES

1. Make sure the parent has answered all questions and has checked the concern column as necessary. If all questions have been answered, go to Step 2. If not all questions have been answered, you should first try to contact the parent to obtain answers or, if necessary, calculate an average score (see pages 39 and 41 of *The ASQ:SE User's Guide*).

2. Review any parent comments. If there are no comments, go to Step 3. If a parent has written in a response, see the section titled "Parent Comments" on pages 39, 41, and 42 of *The ASQ:SE User's Guide* to determine if the response indicates a behavior that may be of concern.

3. Using the following point system:

   Z (for zero) next to the checked box   = 0 points
   V (for Roman numeral V) next to the checked box   = 5 points
   X (for Roman numeral X) next to the checked box   = 10 points
   Checked concern   = 5 points

   Add together:
   | | |
   Total points on page 3   = _25_
   Total points on page 4   = _25_
   Total points on page 5   = _15_
   Total points on page 6   = _15_

   Child's total score = _80_

SCORE INTERPRETATION

1. *Review questionnaires*
   Review the parent's answers to questions. Give special consideration to any individual questions that score 10 or 15 points and any written or verbal comments that the parent shares. Offer guidance, support, and information to families, and refer if necessary, as indicated by score and referral considerations.

2. *Transfer child's total score*
   In the table below, enter the child's total score (transfer total score from above).

Questionnaire interval	Cutoff score	Child's ASQ:SE score
30 months	57	80

3. *Referral criteria*
   Compare the child's total score with the cutoff in the table above. If the child's score falls above the cutoff and the factors in Step 4 have been considered, refer the child for a mental health evaluation.

4. *Referral considerations*
   It is always important to look at assessment information in the context of other factors influencing a child's life. Consider the following variables prior to making referrals for a mental health evaluation. Refer to pages 44–46 in *The ASQ:SE User's Guide* for additional guidance related to these factors and for suggestions for follow-up.

   • Setting/time factors
     (e.g., Is the child's behavior the same at home as at school? Have there been any stressful events in the child's life recently?)
   • Development factors
     (e.g., Is the child's behavior related to a developmental stage or a developmental delay?)
   • Health factors
     (e.g., Is the child's behavior related to health or biological factors?)
   • Family/cultural factors
     (e.g., Is the child's behavior acceptable given cultural or family context?)

Ages & Stages Questionnaires: Social-Emotional, Squires et al.
© 2002 Paul H. Brookes Publishing Co.

7

ASQ:SE   **30 months**

Juanita's return to work, combined with her mother's illness, has caused a lot of stress for the family. John's problems at child care have increased Juanita's stress. Juanita worries about John while she is at work and is feeling overwhelmed. Both Lois and Juanita are guessing that the recent change in setting has been difficult for John and most likely is the cause of his problem behaviors.

Follow-Up

Lois discussed the results of the ASQ:SE with Juanita and Manuel, and together they decided that rather than refer John for a mental health evaluation at this point, they will try to help John become more comfortable in his child care setting and wait a short period of time to see if their interventions are effective. The child care is small, in a home, with 6 children. The child care provider is eager to help John become more comfortable there. Juanita, Manuel, and Lois decided to try the following prior to referral:

- Lois will go to John's child care setting again and observe him. At this point, Lois did not want to rule out the appropriateness of this setting for John. Lois hoped that by observing the setting and the caregiver's interactions with John, she may be able to provide some suggestions to help John feel more comfortable and settled. Lois is going to complete the Family Day Care Rating Scale (Harms & Cryer, 1989; see Appendix E) to look at different aspects of the child care environment that may be affecting John's behavior.

- Lois plans on talking to the child care provider about some of the behaviors John exhibits in child care such as not following directions and having a hard time with transitions between activities. These behaviors may be a result of John's communication difficulties. Some ideas Lois has considered include having an older child interpret directions for John, using picture cues to help John anticipate transitions, and making sure John is given a warning prior to transitions. Lois would like to share her ideas and learn what ideas the child care provider may have.

- One thing that was apparent through discussions with Juanita was that the drop-off time was extremely rushed and always hard for John. Lois talked with her about how important it is to ease into a new routine. Manuel will feed John and help him get dressed before leaving for work. Juanita decided she will leave the house 10–15 minutes earlier so that she can spend some time with John in his child care setting, getting him settled into an activity, before she goes to work.

- Juanita, Manuel, and Lois talked about John's favorite books and activities and about making a tape of John's favorite songs to share with John's child care provider. John's child care provider agreed to call Juanita and Manuel once a week to talk about how John is doing. Juanita suggested that their oldest daughter Rosa might enjoy coming to the child care setting after school a couple of days a week. Juanita thinks John would enjoy having his sister there.

- Juanita and Manuel are going to make an appointment to talk to John's primary health care provider about his throwing up when upset and her concerns about his choking on food. Lois encouraged Juanita and Manuel to ask the health care provider for a referral to a feeding specialist who may be able to provide more guidance in that area.

Lois, Juanita and Manuel, and John's child care provider are going to monitor John's behavior over the next month to see if their ideas make a difference. If John's behavior continues to be a problem or intensifies, they will meet to consider other strategies or a possible referral to a specialist.

NICKY, 16 MONTHS OLD

Nicky is a 16-month-old child who lives with her 14-year-old teenage mother, Lucy; her maternal grandmother, Mona; and an uncle who is 17. The family lives in a small apartment in a city in a midwestern state. Mona works at a grocery store, and Lucy is a freshman in high school.

Soon after Lucy gave birth at home, she abandoned her baby at a church. Fortunately, the baby was found and immediately taken into custody of child protective services. A week later, Lucy told a counselor at school what she had done, and she began the process of trying to regain custody of her daughter. Lucy worked hard to regain custody; she visited regularly with her daughter and completed all of the steps necessary to regain her. Nicky was returned to Lucy under her mother's supervision after 12 months in foster care at a relative's house.

Currently Nicky and Lucy are enrolled in an Early Head Start program where Nicky receives full-day child care. Lucy comes to the Early Head Start center and attends a parenting and child development class for an hour each morning. Lucy spends an additional hour in the center with Nicky and then goes to high school for the rest of the day. Lucy and Mona completed the 18 month ASQ:SE (see the completed questionnaire in Figure D3) during a home visit from an Early Head Start staff person. Nicky received a score of 65 points, 10 points above the cutoff of 55.

Setting/Time Factors

The ASQ:SE shown in Figure D3, completed by Lucy and Mona, primarily reflects Nicky's behavior in the home environment. Nicky's primary caregiver at Early Head Start also completed an ASQ:SE on Nicky, and her responses totaled 95 points. Early Head Start staff mentioned concerns about Nicky being "fussy" and being difficult to console once she gets upset.

Developmental Factors

While she was in foster care, Nicky received early intervention services. She was eligible for Part C early intervention services due to mild delays

Please read each question carefully and
1. Check the box ☐ that best describes your child's behavior *and*
2. Check the circle ○ if this behavior is a concern

	MOST OF THE TIME	SOMETIMES	RARELY OR NEVER	CHECK IF THIS IS A CONCERN
1. Does your child look at you when you talk to him?	☑ z	☐ v	☐ x	○
2. When you leave, does your child remain upset and cry for more than an hour?	☐ x	☑ v 5	☐ z	○
3. Does your child laugh or smile when you play with her?	☑ z	☐ v	☐ x	○
4. Does your child look for you when a stranger approaches?	☑ z	☐ v	☐ x	○
5. Is your child's body relaxed?	☑ z	☐ v	☐ x	○
6. Does your child like to be hugged or cuddled?	☑ z	☐ v	☐ x	○
7. When upset, can your child calm down within 15 minutes?	☐ z	☑ v 5	☐ x	○
8. Does your child stiffen and arch his back when picked up?	☐ x	☑ v 5	☐ z	○
9. Does your child cry, scream, or have tantrums for long periods of time?	☑ x 10	☐ v	☐ z	○

TOTAL POINTS ON PAGE 25

Ages & Stages Questionnaires: Social-Emotional; Squires et al.
© 2002 Paul H. Brookes Publishing Co.

3

ASQ:SE 18 months

	MOST OF THE TIME	SOMETIMES	RARELY OR NEVER	CHECK IF THIS IS A CONCERN
10. Is your child interested in things around her, such as people, toys, and foods?	☑ z	☐ v	☐ x	○
11. Does your child do things over and over and can't seem to stop? Examples are rocking, hand flapping, spinning, or _____ (You may write in something else.)			☐ x	○
12. Does your child have eating problems, such as stuffing foods, vomiting, eating nonfood items, or _____? (You may write in another problem.)	☑ x 10	☐ v	☐ z	○
13. Does your child have trouble falling asleep at naptime or at night?	☑ x 10	☐ v	☐ z	○
14. Do you and your child enjoy mealtimes together?	☑ z	☐ v	☐ x	○
15. Does your child sleep at least 10 hours in a 24-hour period?	☑ z	☐ v	☐ x	○
16. When you point at something, does your child look in the direction you are pointing?	☑ z	☐ v	☐ x	○
17. Does your child get constipated or have diarrhea?	☐ x	☑ v 5	☐ z	○

TOTAL POINTS ON PAGE 35

Ages & Stages Questionnaires: Social-Emotional; Squires et al.
© 2002 Paul H. Brookes Publishing Co.

4

ASQ:SE 18 months

(continued)

Figure D3.   18 month ASQ:SE for Nicky, who is 16 months old. Nicky's mother Lucy and maternal grandmother Mona completed this ASQ:SE.

Figure D3. (continued)

Page 5

	MOST OF THE TIME	SOMETIMES	RARELY OR NEVER	CHECK IF THIS IS A CONCERN
18. Does your child let you know how she is feeling with gestures or words? For example, does she let you know when she is hungry, hurt, or tired?	☑ z	☐ v	☐ x	○
19. Does your child follow simple directions? For example, does he sit down when asked?	☑ z	☐ v	☐ x	○
20. Does your child like to play near or be with family members and friends?	☑ z	☐ v	☐ x	○
21. Does your child check to make sure you are near when exploring new places, such as a park or a friend's home?	☑ z	☐ v	☐ x	○
22. Does your child like to hear stories or sing songs?	☑ z	☐ v	☐ x	○
23. Does your child hurt herself on purpose?	☐ x	☐ v	☑ z	○
24. Does your child like to be around other children?	☑ z	☐ v	☐ x	○
25. Does your child try to hurt other children, adults, or animals (for example, by kicking or biting)?	☐ x	☑ v 5	☐ z	○

TOTAL POINTS ON PAGE 5

Page 6

	MOST OF THE TIME	SOMETIMES	RARELY OR NEVER	CHECK IF THIS IS A CONCERN
26. Has anyone expressed concerns about your child's behaviors? If you checked "sometimes" or "most of the time," please explain:	☐ x	☐ v	☑ z	○

27. Do you have concerns about your child's eating or sleeping behaviors? If so, please explain:
_No_

28. Is there anything that worries you about your child? If so, please explain:
_No_

29. What things do you enjoy most about your child?
She's cute and smart.

TOTAL POINTS ON PAGE 0

18 Month ASQ:SE Information Summary

Child's name: _Nicky Jefferson_   Child's date of birth: _5-15-01_

Person filling out the ASQ:SE: _Lucy & Mona Jefferson_   Relationship to child: _Mother & grandmother_

Mailing address: _17 W. Stony Run Circle_   City: _Cascade_   State: _MI_   ZIP: _____

Telephone: _555-4066_   Assisting in ASQ:SE completion: _____

Today's date: _9-20-01_   Administering program/provider: _Cascade EHS_

SCORING GUIDELINES

1. Make sure the parent has answered all questions and has checked the concern column as necessary. If all questions have been answered, go to Step 2. If not all questions have been answered, you should first try to contact the parent to obtain answers or, if necessary, calculate an average score (see pages 39 and 41 of *The ASQ:SE User's Guide*).

2. Review any parent comments. If there are no comments, go to Step 3. If a parent has written in a response, see the section titled "Parent Comments" on pages 39, 41, and 42 of *The ASQ:SE User's Guide* to determine if the response indicates a behavior that may be of concern.

3. Using the following point system:

Z (for zero) next to the checked box	= 0 points
V (for Roman numeral V) next to the checked box	= 5 points
X (for Roman numeral X) next to the checked box	= 10 points
Checked concern	= 5 points

   Add together:

Total points on page 3	= _25_
Total points on page 4	= _35_
Total points on page 5	= _5_
Total points on page 6	= _0_
Child's total score =	_65_

SCORE INTERPRETATION

1. *Review questionnaires*
   Review the parent's answers to questions. Give special consideration to any individual questions that score 10 or 15 points and any written or verbal comments that parent shares. Offer guidance, support, and information to families, and refer if necessary, as indicated by score and referral considerations.

2. *Transfer child's total score*
   In the table below, enter the child's total score (transfer total score from above).

Questionnaire interval	Cutoff score	Child's ASQ:SE score
18 months	55	65

3. *Referral criteria*
   Compare the child's total score with the cutoff in the table above. If the child's score falls above the cutoff and the factors in Step 4 have been considered, refer the child for a mental health evaluation.

4. *Referral considerations*
   It is always important to look at assessment information in the context of other factors influencing a child's life. Consider the following variables prior to making referrals for a mental health evaluation. Refer to pages 44–46 in *The ASQ:SE User's Guide* for additional guidance related to these factors and for suggestions for follow-up.

   - Setting/time factors
     (e.g., Is the child's behavior the same at home as at school? Have there been any stressful events in the child's life recently?)
   - Development factors
     (e.g., Is the child's behavior related to a developmental stage or a developmental delay?)
   - Health factors
     (e.g., Is the child's behavior related to health or biological factors?)
   - Family/cultural factors
     (e.g., Is the child's behavior acceptable given cultural or family context?)

Ages & Stages Questionnaires: Social-Emotional, Squires et al.
© 2002 Paul H. Brookes Publishing Co.

7

ASQ:SE   **18 months**

145

in her overall development and professional judgment regarding her risk for developmental delays. At 12 months she had made progress, was developmentally on target, was stable in her foster home, and had "graduated" from early intervention services.

Health Factors

Nicky was born 8 weeks premature and weighed 4 pounds, 6 ounces. When Nicky entered foster care, her foster mother reported that she was difficult to feed, had to be rocked to sleep, and woke frequently. By 8 months Nicky had become easier to feed but still woke frequently at night. Nicky was taken to a well-baby checkup at 12 months and has been generally healthy, aside from some colds and ear infections.

Family/Cultural Factors

The recent change in setting is a potential stress factor for Nicky. Nicky's foster care provider is a relative of the family who had offered her home when she heard from Mona about Nicky and Lucy. However, very little was done to prepare or ease the transition for Nicky from foster care to her mother's home.

Follow-Up

With Lucy's consent, the staff at Early Head Start want to have Nicky evaluated for early intervention services—this time for social-emotional concerns. While the staff feel that Nicky's behavior may still be affected by her transition from foster care to her new home, they would like to have a mental health specialist involved. The staff have not seen an improvement in Nicky's behaviors even though she has been in her new home for 4 months (and in consistent child care at the Early Head Start site). The staff have concerns about Lucy's interactions with Nicky and about Lucy's general mental health. The staff are struggling with Nicky's behaviors in child care and would like to get a second opinion. If Nicky is not eligible for early intervention services, the Early Head Start staff hope that they can get some guidance from a specialist about the best way to support Lucy and Nicky. In addition to a referral to a mental health specialist, the Early Head Start staff and Lucy plan to do the following:

- Refer Nicky to her primary health care provider to determine if a biological/health factor might be influencing her behavior.
- Talk to Nicky's former foster mother about Nicky's behaviors. The staff want to encourage the foster mother to visit Nicky and Lucy in the child care center and at home, an option Lucy is happy with. It is hoped that the foster mother may have suggestions about ways to soothe Nicky or may suggest activities that may help ease the transition between foster care and Nicky's new home.

Resources

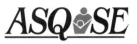

For information on social-emotional screening and assessment tools, see Table 2 in Chapter 2, pages 10–11.

DEVELOPMENTAL SCREENING TOOLS

Ages & Stages Questionnaires (ASQ): A Parent-Completed, Child-Monitoring System, Second Edition

Diane Bricker and Jane Squires, with assistance from Linda Mounts, LaWanda Potter, Robert Nickel, Elizabeth Twombly, and Jane Farrell (1999; available from Paul H. Brookes Publishing Co., Post Office Box 10624, Baltimore, MD 21285-0624; 800-638-3775; http://www. brookespublishing.com)

The ASQ is a psychometrically tested tool that uses caregivers to report on their child's development.

Denver II

William K. Frankenburg, J.B. Dodds, P. Archer, B. Bresnick, P. Maschka, N. Edelman, and H. Shapiro (1992; available from Denver Developmental Materials, Post Office Box 371075, Denver, CO 80237-5075; 800-419-4729)

The Denver II is a commonly used professionally completed screening tool (a revision of the Denver Developmental Screening Test, or DDST).

PARENT–CHILD INTERACTION SCALES

Parent–Child Interaction Feeding and Teaching Scales

Katherine Barnard et al. (1994; available from NCAST, University of Washington, Box 357920, Seattle, WA 98195-7920; 206-543-8528; http://www.son.washington.edu/centers/ncast; ncast@u.washington.edu)

These scales, used by the Parent–Child Interaction Program (also called the Nursing Child Assessment Satellite Teaching, or NCAST), consist of in-depth assessment scales that look at parent–child interactions during feeding and teaching. Use of the assessment scales requires training. A companion videotape series, *Keys to Caregiving*, provides information for professionals working with families with newborns.

Facilitating Caregiver–Infant Communication

M. Diane Klein and Margaret Briggs (available from M. Diane Klein, California State University, Los Angeles, Division of Special Education, 5151 State University Drive, Los Angeles, CA 90032; 323-343-4400; Dklein@calstatela.edu)

This parent–child assessment tool is easy to administer and helpful for focusing on areas in which intervention is needed.

Infant–Caregiver Interaction Scale (ICIS)

Leslie Munson and Sam Odom (available from Leslie Munson, Ph.D., Portland State University, Post Office Box 751, Portland, OR 97207; Munson@pdx.edu)

The ICIS looks at both infant and caregiver behaviors during feeding and play interactions, as well as at the environment. The ICIS helps to target areas to focus on during intervention.

ASSESSMENT TOOLS

Home Observation for Measurement of the Environment (HOME)

Bettye Caldwell and Robert H. Bradley (1984; available from Lorraine Coulson, Center for Applied Studies in Education, College of Education, University of Arkansas at Little Rock, 2801 University Avenue, Little Rock, AR 72204-1099; 505-565-7627; http://www.ualr.edu/~crtldept/home4.htm; lrcoulson@ualr.edu)

This assessment instrument looks at the social and physical home environment. Users need to be aware of some of the issues with this tool related to use with different cultures, appropriateness for children with disabilities, and how to use it in a family-centered manner.

Early Childhood Environmental Rating Scale–Revised (ECERS-R)

Thelma Harms, Richard Clifford, and Debby Cryer (1998)

Family Day Care Rating Scale (FDCRS)

Thelma Harms and Debby Cryer (1989)

Infant/Toddler Environmental Rating Scale (ITERS)

Thelma Harms, Debbie Cryer, and Richard Clifford (1990; the ECERS–R, FDCRS, and ITERS are available from Teachers College Press, 1234 Amsterdam Avenue, New York, NY 10027; 212-678-3929)

These assessment instruments are designed to evaluate the quality of settings for young children in early childhood, family day care, and infant-toddler environments.

FUNCTIONAL BEHAVIORAL ASSESSMENTS

LaRocque, M., Brown, S.E., & Johnson, K.L. (2001). Functional behavioral assessments and intervention plans in early intervention settings. *Infants and Young Children, 13*(3), 59–68

This article provides a good overview on functional behavioral assessments as they apply to very young children.

Functional Assessment and Program Development for Problem Behavior: A Practical Handbook, Second Edition

R.E. O'Neil, R.H. Horner, R.W. Albin, J.R. Sprague, K. Storkey, and J.S. Newton (1997; available from Brooks/Cole Thomson Learning, Pacific Grove, CA; http://www.brookscole.com)

CURRICULA/RESOURCES WITH A SOCIAL-EMOTIONAL EMPHASIS

Touchpoints: Your Child's Emotional and Behavioral Development

T. Berry Brazelton (1994; available from Perseus Books, Perseus Books Group Customer Service Department, 5500 Central Avenue, Boulder, CO 80301; http://www.perseuspublishing.com)

Touchpoints is a reference book for parents or professionals on a young child's social-emotional development.

The Creative Curriculum for Infants and Toddlers, Revised Edition

Amy Laura Combro, Laura J. Colker, and Diane Trister Dodge (1999)

The Creative Curriculum for Family Childcare

Diane Trister Dodge and Laura J. Colker (1991)

The Creative Curriculum for Early Childhood, Third Edition

Diane Trister Dodge and Laura J. Colker (1992; these three *Creative Curriculum* books are available from Teaching Strategies, Inc., Post Office Box 42243, Washington, DC 20015; 800-637-3652; http://www. teachingstrategies.com)

These excellent overall curricula place a strong emphasis on creating environments for young children in infant-toddler, family childcare, and early childhood settings.

Partnership in Parenting Education (PIPE)

(1994; available from How to Read Your Baby, 280 Columbine Street, Suite 311, Denver, CO 80206; 303-377-4584; http://www. howtoreadyourbaby.com)

This parenting curriculum focuses on developing a positive emotional relationship between parent and child. Users are encouraged to participate in a training to familiarize with content and implementation of the model.

The Program for Infant/Toddler Caregivers (PITC)

Developed by WestEd in collaboration with the California Department of Education (available from California Department of Education, CDE Press, Sales Office, Post Office Box 271, Sacramento, CA 95812; 800-995-4099; 916-445-1260; http://www.pitc.org)

PITC consists of intensive training sessions on four module topics. The four modules cover the following topics: social-emotional growth and socialization; group care; learning and development; and culture, family, and providers.

ORGANIZATIONS

American Academy of Pediatrics (AAP)

141 Northwest Point Boulevard, Elk Grove Village, IL 60007-1098; 847-434-4000; http://www.aap.org

The AAP offers a variety of materials, including breastfeeding information and brochures; an overview of early emotional development; and the *Pediatric Nutrition Handbook, Fourth Edition.*

Center for Effective Collaboration and Practice

1000 Thomas Jefferson Street, NW, Suite 400, Washington, DC 20007; 888-457-1551; 202-944-5300 http://www.air.org/cecp/

This center can provide in-depth information on functional behavioral assessments.

I Am Your Child

Post Office Box 15605, Beverly Hills, CA 90209; 310-285-2385; *or* 1325 6th Avenue, 30th Floor, New York, NY 10019; 212-636-5030; http://www.iamyourchild.org

National Association for the Education of Young Children (NAEYC)

1509 16th Street, NW, Washington, DC 20036-1426; http://www.naeyc.org

National Early Childhood Technical Assistance System (NEC*TAS)

c/o Frank Porter Graham Child Development Center, University of North Carolina at Chapel Hill, 137 East Franklin Street, Suite 500, Chapel Hill, NC 27514

National Head Start Association

1651 Prince Street, Alexandria, VA 22314; 703-739-0875; http://www.nhsa.org

National Center for Education in Maternal and Child Health (NCEMCH)

2000 15th Street, N., Arlington, VA 22201-2617; 703-524-7802; http://www.ncemch.org

NCEMCH manages the Bright Futures Project (http://www.brightfutures.org), which builds partnerships between health care providers and families.

National Technical Assistance Center for Children's Mental Health

Child Development Center, Georgetown University, 3307 M Street, NW, Washington, DC 20007-3935; 202-687-5000; http://www.georgetown.edu/cassp

Positive Behavioral Interventions and Support Technical Center

Behavioral Research and Training, 5262 University of Oregon, Eugene, OR 97403-5262; 541-346-2505; http://www.pbis.org

ZERO TO THREE: National Center for Infants, Toddlers and Families

2000 M Street, NW, Suite 200, Washington, DC 20036; 202-638-1144; http://zerotothree.org

FURTHER PUBLICATIONS ON THE ASQ:SE

Bricker, D., Davis, M., & Squires, J. (in press). Mental health screening in young children. *Infants and Young Children.*

Squires, J. (2000). Identifying social/emotional and behavioral problems in infants and toddlers. *Infant/Toddler Intervention, 10*(2), 107–119.

Squires, J., Bricker, D., Heo, K., & Twombly, E. (2001). Identification of social-emotional problems in young children using a parent-completed screening measure. *Early Childhood Research Quarterly, 16,* 405–419.

Squires, J., Bricker, D., & Twombly, E. (in press). Parent-completed screening for social emotional problems in young children: Effects of risk/disability status and gender on performance. *Infant Mental Health.*

Squires, J., & Nickel, R. (in press). Never too soon: Identification of social-emotional problems in infants and toddlers. *Contemporary Pediatrics.*

Glossary

This glossary contains definitions of terminology used in this volume to discuss the screening of children.

Average score   Mean score, obtained by adding scores on ASQ:SE items for a total score and then dividing by the number of questions answered. Average score is used in calculating the child's final total score when parents do not answer all questions: total score + (average score × number of questions not answered) = final total score.

Cutoff point   Empirically derived score that indicates the point at which a child's performance begins to be suspect and referral for further assessment is appropriate.

Developmental assessment   Establishes baseline, or entry level of measurement, of a child's skills across developmental areas (e.g., communication, gross motor, fine motor, problem solving, personal-social).

Identified   Also known as *screened*. Descriptive of children whose scores on a screening tool, such as the ASQ:SE, are above the cutoff score and who are identified as needing further assessment.

Median   50th percentile of a distribution; point below which half of the observations fall.

Monitoring   Periodic developmental screening of young children.

Overreferral (or overidentification)   Also known as *overscreening*. The proportion of children incorrectly identified as in need of further assessment by the screening tool.

Percent agreement   The proportion of agreement between the screening tool and standardized assessments or diagnosis.

Percent screened   The percentage of children who are identified as needing further assessment by a screening tool.

Positive predictive value   The probability that a child identified by the screening tool as needing further assessment will have intervention needs.

Psychometric study   Research examining the validity and reliability of an assessment instrument.

Receiver operating characteristic (ROC) curve   Procedure to determine optimal cutoff points on a screening tool. Curves are generated (using a computer program) using potential cutoff points. Cutoff points are then selected that maximize sensitivity (true positives) and specificity (true negatives).

Reliability   Consistency of test scores over time and between testers; the extent to which it is possible to generalize from one test result conducted by one person to test results conducted at different times or by different observers.

Screening   A brief procedure to determine whether a child requires further and more comprehensive evaluation.

Semi-interquartile range   One half of the distance between the first quartile of scores (25% of distribution) and the third quartile (75% of distribution): (Quartile 3 – Quartile 1) ÷ 2.

Sensitivity   The proportion of children correctly identified as needing further assessment by the screening tool and who perform below the expected level on a standardized assessment or assessment battery.

Skewed curve   Asymmetrical distribution in which the majority is very high or very low. The ASQ:SE scores are positively skewed, with the majority of scores between 0 and 25.

Specificity   The proportion of children correctly excluded as developing typically by the screening tool and who perform at the expected level on a standardized assessment.

Tracking   Periodic and sequential developmental screening and referral of young children for intervention services.

Underreferral (or underidentification)   Also known as underscreening. The proportion of children incorrectly identified as developing typically by the screening tool.

Utility   Usefulness; ease of use of the screening tool or procedure.

Validity   Extent to which a test measures what its authors claim it measures; appropriateness of the inferences that can be made on test results.

G

Sample Forms and Letters—Spanish Version
Ejemplos de formularios y cartas—Versión en español

ASQ:SE

Throughout this volume, a number of sample forms, as well as letters to the parents and physicians of children participating in an ASQ:SE monitoring program, are provided. To assist program staff who serve Spanish-speaking families, these samples have been translated into Spanish and are provided in this appendix. Staff are granted permission to photocopy these samples and to modify them to suit the needs of their program and the families they serve. The *Ages & Stages Questionnaires: Social-Emotional* are available in Spanish as well.

A lo largo de este volumen, se provee varios ejemplos de formularios además de ejemplos de cartas a los padres y a los médicos de los niños que participan en el programa del ASQ:SE. Para ayudar a los proveedores del programa que sirven a las familias hispanohablantes, estos formularios y cartas aparecen traducidos en español en este apéndice. Es permitido fotocopiar y modificarlos para mejor acomodar las necesidades individuales del programa y de las familias que sirven. Se puede conseguir los cuestionarios del *Edades y Etapas: Social-Emocional* en español también.

ASQ:SE

Estimados [fill in parents' or guardians' names]:

Los primeros 5 años en la vida de su hijo/a son muy importantes, porque es el período que lo/a preparara para el triunfo escolar y el resto de su vida. Durante su infancia y su niñez, muchas experiencias deben ser adquiridas y muchas nuevas habilidades aprendidas. Es importante asegurarse de que el progreso de desarrollo en cada niño/a avance sin ningún problema durante este período; por eso, estamos interesados en ayudarles seguir el desarrollo social y emocional de su niño/a. Ustedes nos pueden ayudar al completar el siguiente cuestionario que les llegará por correo en intervalos desde 6 a 12 meses. Se les harán preguntas acerca de algunas de las cosas que haga o no haga su niño/a. Por favor devuelva por correo tal cuestionario a [fill in staff member's name].

Si el cuestionario completado nos indica que su niño/a parece estar desarrollándose sin ningún problema, les enviaremos una carta indicándoles que el desarrollo social y emocional de su niño/a parece estar avanzando bien. Entonces al tiempo apropiado les enviaremos el cuestionario del próximo nivel de edad.

Si ustedes tienen alguna preocupación por su niño/a en cualquier momento, puede hablar con un proveedor del programa para discutir sus preocupaciones. Si el cuestionario completado sugiere que haya alguna preocupación por su niño/a, nos pondremos en contacto con usted directamente. Tal vez ustedes querrán que el médico de su niño u otra agencia haga un examen más profundo. Toda información adquirida sobre su niño/a y su familia será mantenida el la confidencia más estricta.

Sinceramente,

[fill in staff member's name]
[fill in program name]

The ASQ:SE User's Guide, Squires, Bricker, and Twombly. © 2002 Paul H. Brookes Publishing Co.
La guía de uso del ASQ:SE, Squires, Bricker y Twombly. © 2002 Paul H. Brookes Publishing Co.

Sample information and agreement letter to parents. This letter should be modified by personnel to reflect the ASQ:SE method(s) to be used by the program.

ASQ:SE

_____ He leido la descripción del proyecto monitorial y deseo participar. Estoy dispuesto/a a completar los cuestionarios acerca del desarrollo de mi niño/a y los devolveré con prontitud.

_____ He leido la descripción del proyecto monitorial. Comprendo el propósito de este programa y no deseo participar.

Firma del padre o la madre o el guardián _____

Fecha _____

Nombre del niño/a _____

Fecha de nacimiento del niño/a _____

Nombre del doctor del niño/a _____

The ASQ:SE User's Guide, Squires, Bricker, and Twombly. © 2002 Paul H. Brookes Publishing Co.
La guía de uso del ASQ:SE, Squires, Bricker y Twombly. © 2002 Paul H. Brookes Publishing Co.

Sample of a participation agreement to be signed by a child's parent or guardian before beginning implementation procedures.

ASQ:SE

Estimados padres:

Quisiéramos que tomasen unos minutos para evaluar nuestro cuestionario. Apreciamos muchísimo su participación en nuestro programa, y esperamos que nuestro servicio les haya ayudado.

1. ¿Fueron apropiados los cuestionarios para su niño/a?

    sí ☐   no ☐

    Comentarios:

2. ¿Fueron útiles los cuestionarios para completar?

    sí ☐   no ☐

    Comentarios:

3. ¿Encontraron ustedes alguna pregunta poco clara o difícil de entender?

    sí ☐   no ☐

    Si ustedes han marcado "sí", ¿cuál?

    Comentarios:

4. ¿A ustedes les gustaría recibir más información sobre el desarrollo social-emocional?

    sí ☐   no ☐

    Si ustedes han marcado "sí", ¿en cuáles áreas?

    Comentarios:

5. ¿Querría usted completar otro cuestionario cuando su niño tenga más edad?

    sí ☐   no ☐

    Comentarios:

Apreciamos cualquier comentario más que ustedes tengan sobre los cuestionarios. Ustedes pueden escribir al revés de esta hoja.

The ASQ:SE User's Guide, Squires, Bricker, and Twombly. © 2002 Paul H. Brookes Publishing Co.
La guía de uso del ASQ:SE, Squires, Bricker y Twombly. © 2002 Paul H. Brookes Publishing Co.

An example of a feedback form. Such a survey should be distributed at least once a year, if possible.

Información de la Familia   ASQ:SE

1. Número de identificación de su hijo/a _____
2. Nombre de su hijo/a _____
   Nombre de los padres (apellido, nombre) _____
3. Su dirrección: Numéro, calle _____
   Ciudad _____
   Condado _____ Estado/Provincia _____ Código/Zona postal _____
   Teléfono: Domicilio_____
   Trabajo _____
4. Fecha de nacimiento (mes, dia, año) _____ / _____ / _____
5. Sexo (hijo = 1, hija = 2) _____
6. Etnicidad de su hijo/a _____
7. Peso del recién nacido (en libras, onzas) _____
8. ¿Necesitaba su bebé cuidado intensivo? (1 = sí, 2 = no) _____
   ¿Por cuánto tiempo? (en días) _____
9. Fecha de entrada en el programa monitorial (mes, día, año) _____ / _____ / _____
10. Estado de su hijo/a:
    ¿A riesgo? (1 = sí, 2 = no) _____
    Si es afirmativa, escriba 3 factores primarios: _____
    ¿Tiene su bebé problemas físicos? (1 = sí, 2 = no) _____
    Incapacidad (apúntelas) _____
11. ¿Es una familia adoptiva? (1 = sí, 2 = no) _____
12. ¿Cuántos años tiene la madre de nacimiento? _____
13. Apellido paternal de la madre: _____
14. ¿Estado marital de la madre? _____
15. ¿Hasta que año completó la madre la escuela? _____
16. ¿Hasta que año completó la pareja la escuela? _____
17. ¿Qué tipo de trabajo hace la madre? _____
18. ¿Qué tipo de trabajo hace la pareja? _____
19. ¿Cuánto ganan al año? _____
20. El médico del niño/a _____
    Teléfono (o nombre de la clínica) _____
21. ¿Tuvo el niño/a cualquier problema médico o de desarollo? _____
    Si es afirmativa, explique _____
22. ¿Cuántos niños viven en su hogar? _____

A sample Child and Family Demographic Information Form. This form or one like it should be easily accessible throughout the child's involvement in the program.

N° de identificación _____

Sumario Informativo del Niño/a

ASQ⋅SE

1. Nombre del niño/a _____
2. Fecha de nacimiento del niño/a (mes, día, año) _____ / _____ / _____
3. Sexo (hijo = 1, hija = 2) _____
4. Nombre del padre, la madre o el guardián (apellido, nombre) _____
5. Otros guardianes _____
6. Domicilio: Numéro, calle _____
   Ciudad _____
   Condado _____ Estado/Provincia _____ Código/Zona postal _____
   Teléfono: Domicilio _____
   Trabajo _____
7. Proveedor primario de los cuidados de la salud _____
   Teléfono (o nombre de la clínica) _____
8. Notas/comentarios _____
   _____
   _____

The ASQ:SE User's Guide, Squires, Bricker, and Twombly. © 2002 Paul H. Brookes Publishing Co.
La guía de uso del ASQ:SE, Squires, Bricker y Twombly. © 2002 Paul H. Brookes Publishing Co.

The Child Information Summary Form should be completed during the first step of the implementation phase. It should be kept in the child's file.

ASQ⋅SE

Estimados [fill in parents' or guardians' names]:

Gracias por completar el cuestionario del *Edades y Etapas: Social-Emocional* para su hijo/a. Sus respuestas en el cuestionario indican que el desarollo de su hijo/a parece estar avanzando bien.

Otro cuestionario será enviado a ustedes en [fill in number here] meses. Favor de recordar otra vez la importancia de completar todas las preguntas y devolver el cuestionario tan pronto como sea posible. Favor de llamarnos si ustedes tienen alguna pregunta. Gracias por su interés en nuestro programa.

¡Muchas gracias!

[fill in staff member's name]
[fill in program name]

The ASQ:SE User's Guide, Squires, Bricker, and Twombly. © 2002 Paul H. Brookes Publishing Co.
La guía de uso del ASQ:SE, Squires, Bricker y Twombly. © 2002 Paul H. Brookes Publishing Co.

A sample feedback letter to parents or guardians whose children's ASQ:SE scores indicate typical development.

Index

Page references followed by *t* indicate tables; those followed by *f* indicate figures.

Please send me

ASQ set (ASQ User's Guide plus Questionnaires)
_____ Stock #370X / $190.00— with Questionnaires in English
_____ Stock #3718 / $190.00—with Questionnaires in Spanish
_____ Stock #4838 / $190.00—with Questionnaires in French
_____ Stock #5273 / $140.00—with Questionnaires in Korean (Korean questionnaires are available for use at 4, 6, 8, 12, 16, 18, 20, 24, 30, 36, and 48 months.)

ASQ CD-ROM
_____ Stock #6938 / $190.00—in English
_____ Stock #6954 / $190.00—in Spanish

ASQ Questionnaires
_____ Stock #3688 / $165.00—in English
_____ Stock #3696 / $165.00—in Spanish
_____ Stock #482X / $165.00—in French
_____ Stock #8015 / $115.00—in Korean

ASQ questionnaires are available in other languages. For more information call **1-800-638-3775.**

The ASQ User's Guide, _Second Edition_
_____ Stock #367X / $45.00—in English

Ages & Stages Questionnaires on a Home Visit (video)
_____ Stock #2185 / $44.00—in English

· ·

___ Check enclosed (payable to Brookes Publishing Co.)

___ Purchase Order attached (bill my institution)

___ Please charge my credit card: ○ American Express   ○ MasterCard   ○ Visa

Credit Card #: _____   Exp. Date: _____

Signature (required with credit card use): _____

Name: _____ Daytime Phone: _____

Street Address: _____ ❏ residential ❏ commercial
Complete street address required.

City/State/ZIP: _____   Country: _____

E-mail Address: _____
❏ Yes! I want to receive special web site discount offers! My e-mail address will not be shared with any other party.

Photocopy this form, and mail it to **Brookes Publishing Co.,** P.O. Box 10624, Baltimore, MD 21285-0624, U.S.A.;
FAX **410-337-8539;** Call **1-800-638-3775** (8 A.M.–5 P.M., ET U.S.A. and CAN) or **410-337-9580** (worldwide);
or order online at **www.brookespublishing.com**

Shipping & Handling			Shipping rates are for UPS Ground Delivery within continental U.S.A. For other shipping options and rates, call 1-800-638-3775 (in the U.S.A. and CAN) and 410-337-9580 (worldwide).
For pretax total of	Add*	For CAN	
$0.00 - $49.99	$5.00	$7.00	
$50.00 - $69.99	10%	$7.00	
$70.00 - $399.99	10%	10%	
$400.00 and over	8%	8%	
*calculate percentage on product total			

Subtotal $ _____

5% sales tax, Maryland only +$ _____

7% business tax (GST), CAN only +$ _____

Shipping (see chart) +$ _____

Total (in U.S.A. dollars) =$ _____

Your list code is **BA 113**

All prices in U.S.A. dollars. Policies and prices subject to change without notice. Prices may be higher outside the U.S.A. You may return books within 30 days for a full credit of the product price. Refunds will be issued for prepaid orders. Items must be returned in resalable condition.

Ages & Stages Questionnaires

A Parent Completed, Child-Monitoring System, *Second Edition*

By Diane Bricker, Ph.D., & Jane Squires, Ph.D.,
with assistance from Linda Mounts, M.A., LaWanda Potter, M.S.,
Robert Nickel, M.D., Elizabeth Twombly, M.S., & Jane Farrell, M.S.

With the ASQ, professionals will be able to assess skills in five developmental areas:

- communication
- gross motor
- fine motor
- problem solving
- personal-social

Just like the **ASQ:SE,** parents complete the short, simple questionnaires. Then, in just a minute's time, professionals convert parents' responses of **yes**, **sometimes**, and **not yet** to color-coded scoring sheets, enabling them to quickly determine a child's progress in each developmental area. It's a flexible, reliable, and economical way to track the developmental progress of young children.

ASQ comes with 19 color-coded, reproducible questionnaires for use at 4, 6, 8, 10, 12, 14, 16, 18, 20, 22, 24, 27, 30, 33, 36, 42, 48, 54, and 60 months of age, and 19 reproducible, age-appropriate scoring sheets—1 for each questionnaire.

NOW AVAILABLE IN TWO FORMATS!

- **ASQ Boxed Questionnaires** include all 19 questionnaires, all 19 scoring sheets, and a reproducible mail-back sheet for questionnaires, all in one convenient storage box.

- **ASQ CD-ROM** contains all 19 questionnaires, all 19 scoring sheets, **PLUS** all 200 intervention activities from the **ASQ User's Guide,** in English or Spanish. All materials are in PDF format for easy printing and photocopying at no additional cost.

Additional ASQ components:

- **ASQ User's Guide, *Second Edition.*** The User's Guide has been revised and expanded to help professionals accurately administer the questionnaires and confidently interpret their results. Sample parent-child activities for each age range are included.

- **The Ages & Stages Questionnaires on a Home Visit.** This instructive video shows professionals how to conduct **ASQ** on home visits, with firsthand footage of a home visitor guiding a family with three children through the items on a questionnaire.

PLACE YOUR ORDER NOW—

fill out the order form on the back of this page and mail today!

ASQ:SE Order Form

Please send me

The Complete ASQ:SE (User's Guide plus Questionnaires)
_____ Stock #5346 / $125.00—with Questionnaires in English
_____ Stock #5370 / $125.00—with Questionnaires in Spanish

ASQ:SE Questionnaires
_____ Stock #532X / $100.00—in English
_____ Stock #5362 / $100.00—in Spanish

The ASQ:SE User's Guide
_____ Stock #5338 / $40.00—in English

· ·

___ Check enclosed (payable to Brookes Publishing Co.)

___ Purchase Order attached (bill my institution)

___ Please charge my credit card: ○ American Express   ○ MasterCard   ○ Visa

Credit Card #: _____   Exp. Date: _____

Signature (required with credit card use): _____

Name: _____Daytime Phone: _____

Street Address: _____ ❏ residential ❏ commercial
Complete street address required.

City/State/ZIP: _____   Country: _____

E-mail Address: _____
❏ Yes! I want to receive special web site discount offers! My e-mail address will not be shared with any other party.

Photocopy this form, and mail it to **Brookes Publishing Co.,** P.O. Box 10624, Baltimore, MD 21285-0624, U.S.A.;
FAX **410-337-8539;** Call **1-800-638-3775** (8 A.M.–5 P.M., ET U.S.A. and CAN) or **410-337-9580** (worldwide);
or order online at **www.brookespublishing.com**

Shipping & Handling		
For pretax total of	Add*	For CAN
$0.00 - $49.99	$5.00	$7.00
$50.00 - $69.99	10%	$7.00
$70.00 - $399.99	10%	10%
$400.00 and over	8%	8%
*calculate percentage on product total		

Shipping rates are for UPS Ground Delivery within continental U.S.A. For other shipping options and rates, call 1-800-638-3775 (in the U.S.A. and CAN) and 410-337-9580 (worldwide).

All prices in U.S.A. dollars. Policies and prices subject to change without notice. Prices may be higher outside the U.S.A. You may return books within 30 days for a full credit of the product price. Refunds will be issued for prepaid orders. Items must be returned in resalable condition.

Subtotal $ _____

5% sales tax, Maryland only⁺ $ _____

7% business tax (GST), CAN only⁺ $ _____

Shipping (see chart)⁺ $ _____

Total (in U.S.A. dollars)= $ _____

Your list code is **BA 113**

· ·

Browse our entire catalog, read excerpts, and find special offers at
www.brookespublishing.com